面向国际的
中西医结合防治新型冠状病毒肺炎
诊疗建议方案

Diagnosis and Treatment Protocol for COVID-19
An Integrated Approach Combining Chinese and Western Medicine
Recommended for International Community

（汉英对照）

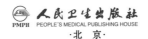

人民卫生出版社
PMPH PEOPLE'S MEDICAL PUBLISHING HOUSE
·北 京·

寄　语

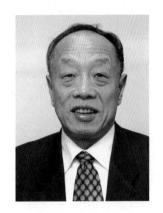

李肇星

中华人民共和国外交部前部长

中国民族医药学会国际交流与合作分会名誉会长

交流互鉴，人类共享

院士评述

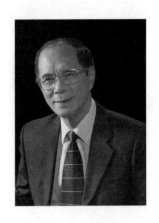

北京大学神经科学研究所名誉所长

中国科学院院士

中医药是源于中华民族的健康宝库，针灸的应用历史已有2 000多年，对于动员机体自身抗病物质有良好作用，对急慢性功能性疾病，及重病康复阶段有积极意义。

在新冠肺炎全球肆虐的今日，我们同世界人民一样感同身受，我们愿把一线专家中西医结合抗击疫情的宝贵经验奉献出来和世界人民共享，为构建人类命运共同体出一份力量。

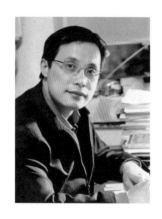

中国中医科学院院长

中国工程院院士

国家援武汉首批中医医疗队领队

　　新冠肺炎疫情危及全球人民生命安全，中国政府在新冠肺炎防治中的成功举措和经验应与人类共享。编制让国际同仁"看得懂、用得上"的中西医结合防治新冠肺炎传染病的诊疗方案势在必行。本方案充分汇总了我国治疗新冠肺炎的经验和成果，根据疫情分期、分型治疗。每一个分型都有基础方、根据伴随症状随症加减。整个方案全面、有效且易懂、易操作，值得推广实施，并在具体实施中根据出现的问题不断修订、优化，使其更加科学、普适，惠及人类。

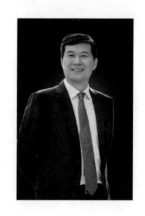

清华大学临床医学院院长

北京清华长庚医院院长

中国工程院院士

新冠肺炎全球蔓延，给世界各国人民的生命和健康带来严重危机。目前，对于人类尚未认识的病毒性传染病尚无有效的药物治疗。在此情形下，中医在病人照护中可带来一定价值。让我们携手合作为全球抗疫做出贡献！

国际专家评述

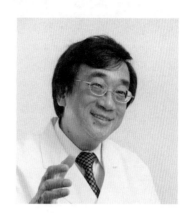

内田俊也

日本帝京平成大学国际交流中心主任

帝京大学医学部前部长

　　该方案无论是对医务工作者，还是对基层医生，为他们挽救患者，都提供了极大的帮助。

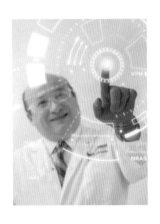

Horacio Astudillo de la Vega

纽约科学院院士、墨西哥国家科学技术委员会顾问和评价委员
墨西哥社会保障研究所（IMSS）21 世纪国家医学中心肿瘤转化研究
与细胞治疗实验室研究员

"该病毒的病理和感染潜力很大，目前几乎没有病毒制剂显示对其有杀伤力。在已有的解释的基础上，今天我们可以考虑一种对生理致病机制的新解释，我们也必须考虑它，才能在这类患者中实现充分的治疗反应。2019-CoV 感染患者的肺血栓形成可能诱导内皮功能障碍和血栓前间质性炎症带来的损伤，然后通过补体和细胞因子的释放和凝血激活，伴随毛细血管和肺泡微血栓形成，导致严重的急性炎症，同时诱发局部消耗性凝血病，即弥散性血管内凝血（DIC），这就是急性呼吸窘迫综合征（ARDS）的成因。"他特别强调了一些中药的参与模式，"我们必须综合用药，以减少伴随抗凝治疗的细胞因子诱导的炎症反应，从而改善内皮功能，挽救这些患者已经严重受损的气体交换功能。"

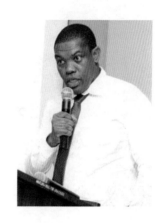

Liggyle 教授

坦桑尼亚卫生部公共卫生负责人

中医中药博大精深，令人赞叹不已！该治疗方案需要根据辨证分型，采用不同种类的药材并特殊熬制，若能直接提供药物，更多人会乐意接受。

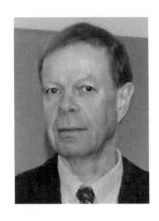

C G Östenson

瑞典卡罗林斯卡皇家医学院高级教授

　　目前全球健康状况令人担忧，对于中西医结合治疗我们也非常感兴趣。同时，对中国医疗同行的不遗余力表示感谢。

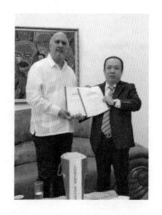

卡洛斯·米格尔·佩雷拉

古巴驻华大使

我对中国抗击疫情取得的成绩表示赞赏和钦佩，认为中国民族医药学会国际交流与合作分会送来的诊疗建议方案及时、珍贵。希望下一步双方积极开展防疫合作，共同推动古巴生物医学和中国中西医在防治研究时交换信息，并在两国医疗团队到第三方国家抗疫防疫时进行交流合作。

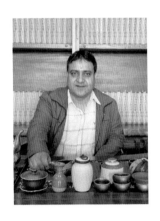

Prakash Gyawali 教授

尼泊尔替代医学（非西医）部健康促进科负责人
临床心理学家和公共卫生专家、尼泊尔阿育吠陀医师协会主席

　　众所周知，中国在抗击新冠病毒中做出了非同凡响的成就。该方案在抗击新冠病毒方面非常实用。尽管在诊疗方案中，有很多是草药，但要在我们国家推行该诊疗方案应会行之有效。

目　录

Contents

新冠肺炎传染病疫情对世界人民生命安全和身体健康带来重大威胁，也对世界卫生事业构成严重挑战。疫情暴发以来，中国政府在习近平主席亲自指挥部署下，采取得力措施控制疫情蔓延，目前中国国内疫情防控形势仍旧严峻复杂。世界卫生组织总干事谭德塞指出，中国强有力的举措不仅是在保护中国人民，也是在保护世界人民，为全球疫情防控赢得了时间。

在习近平主席领导下，中国政府卫生行政部门运用中西医结合开展疫情防治，取得积极有效成果。中医药是中西医结合的重要组成部分，是中华民族的瑰宝，有着源远流长的历史，在中华民族数千年的发展过程中帮助中国人战胜过无数次大瘟大疫。2003年的非典疫情，以及近两个月中国抗击新冠肺炎疫情中中医药都显示出很好的疗效，在现代科技的支撑下，与西医紧密合作，发挥了独特作用，中医药对不同阶段不同症状的患者都得到有效应用。根据3月23日中国国务院新闻办公室新闻发布会和国家中医药管理局负责人余艳红介绍：中国确诊病例中有74 187人使用了中医药治疗，占总数91.5%；湖北有61 449名患者使用了中医药治疗，占90.6%。临床疗效观察显示，中医药总有效率达到90%以上，中药干预组轻症患者病情无一加重；使用中药汤药组的重型/危重型患者死亡风险降低八成多；中药干预组复阳率约为2.77%，而没有无中药干预组的复阳率为15.79%。中国中西医结合方案从安全性、有效性、适用性、经济性等方面都具备向全球推广使用的条件。

在中国政府及国家中医药管理局的倡议下，为服务人类命运共同体建设和促进国际防疫合作，增强国际医学界对中国中西医结合方案的理解，根据中国的有效经验，中国民族医药学会国际交流与合作分会积极响应，秉承交流互鉴、人类共享，打造健康命运共同体的立会宗旨，设立专项课题，由中国中医科学院、清华大学附属北京清华长庚医院、江西中医药大学、北京中医药大学、原309医院等单位的中医温病学、传染病医院管理、药理、制剂、翻译、对外交流方面的高级别知名专家组成的研究团队，根据中国新冠肺炎武汉国家中医医疗队和代表性省份的一线专家临床实践经验，参照中国国家卫生健康委和国家中医药管理局颁布的《新型冠状病毒感染的肺炎诊疗方案》及中国各省颁布的新型冠状病毒感染的肺炎中医药防治方案，结合当前国际新型冠状病毒感染的肺炎的具体临床症状和相关国际法规，平行征求日本、瑞典、古巴、坦桑尼亚、墨西哥等国的医学专家意见，形成了力争让国际同仁"看得懂、用得上"的《面向国际的中西医结合防治新型冠状病毒肺炎诊疗建议方案》。

中医用药的原则是"三因制宜"（因时、因地、因人），课题组将根据本方案国际合作的进展，结合应用国的具体情况和需求，持续修订优化版本。

守望相助、共克时艰是我们的初衷，彼此信赖、相互合作是我们的期望。我们愿同国际同仁携手同行，共同努力，赢得这场人类同重大传染性疾病的伟大斗争！

一、方案编撰背景和基本思路

本方案的编撰思路是，面向国际，中西医紧密结合，发挥优势，互相支持。方案通过挖掘中国数千年防治疫病的历史文献，结合现代医学研究成果，充分体现中西医深度融合。借鉴中国国家卫生健康委和国家中医药管理局《新型冠状病毒感染的肺炎诊疗方案》及全国各省颁布的新型冠状病毒感染的肺炎中医药防治方案，具有理论依据、临床经验和实际操作效果。

二、方案的主要特点

（一）语言通用，表述统一。从传统中医药语系转化为现代医学表述方式，从中文转译为国际通用语言，用统一的语言体系，使中医认可、西医能懂，充分发挥中西医结合的效能。

（二）分阶段、模块，体例简明。为了适合国际各国的理解和操作，按疫情分成预防、疑似、轻型与普通型、重型、危重型、恢复期六个阶段，每阶段一个基础方，根据具体不同症状，采用中成药联合辨证用药，形成模块化、表单化，达到方便、有效、易懂、易操作的目的。

（三）三因制宜，有的放矢。为了便于准确诊断，因人因地因时施药，方案设计了远程舌诊采集和问诊采集表，详细了解掌握患者的具体症状，达到有的放矢，针对性强，提升效果。

（四）遵循历史经典，坚持科学标准。一是处方以中医经典古方为主，有长期应用历史和确切效果，积累了大量真实世界证据（Real World Evidence，RWE），又有中华人民共和国药典（2020年版）、中华人民共和国原卫生部药品标准依据。二是剂型适用方便。首先选择片剂、胶囊、颗粒剂、口服液，其次是传统丸剂、煮散剂，既保障临床效果，又关注患者接受程度。三是药材原料合规。考虑各国法规要求，汤剂规避有安全隐患的禁用、慎用药材（如麻黄、细辛等），不用濒危、野生动植物，保证合法、合规。

（五）中外专家合作，体现共同智慧。方案编制团队组织结构体现了中医与西医结合、医学与药学结合、多学科结合、老中青结合，既有一线实战经验丰富的临床专家，也有德高望重的国家级名老中医指导，同时，与全球五大洲的医药专家代表进行充分交流、研讨，体现国际专家共同意见。

三、方案编制和国际分享组织架构

（一）方案编撰指导

黄璐琦　中国中医科学院院长，中国工程院院士

董家鸿　中国清华大学临床医学院院长、北京清华长庚医院院长，中国
　　　　　工程院院士

（二）国际分享

黄桂芳　中国民族医药学会国际交流与合作分会副会长，中国国务院外
　　　　　事办公室前副主任、国务院办公厅秘书局前局长，中国驻菲律
　　　　　宾、新西兰、津巴布韦前大使

徐贻聪　中国驻古巴、阿根廷、厄瓜多尔前大使，中国外交部拉美司前副司长

郭崇立　中国民族医药学会国际交流与合作分会副会长，中国外交部新闻司前副司长、中国驻牙买加、肯尼亚前大使，中国驻联合国环境署、人居署前代表

赵荣宪　中国民族医药学会国际交流与合作分会副会长，中国外交部拉美司前副司长，中国驻古巴、委内瑞拉前大使

吴思科　中国外交部外交政策咨询委员会委员，中国民族医药学会国际交流与合作分会咨询委员，中国外交部西亚北非司前司长，中国驻埃及、沙特前大使、中国中东特使

周晓沛　中国民族医药学会国际交流与合作分会咨询委员，中国外交部欧亚司前司长、中国驻乌克兰、波兰、哈萨克斯坦前大使

傅元聪　中国民族医药学会国际交流与合作分会咨询委员，中国外交部前驻东帝汶特命全权大使

（三）中医审定

刘景源　中国国家级名老中医，北京中医药大学教授、博士生导师，中医温病学家

（四）英文定稿

陈明明　中国民族医药学会国际交流与合作分会主任委员，中国外交部公共外交咨询委员，中国外交部翻译室前主任，中国驻新西兰、瑞典前大使

（五）总策划

杨　凯　中国民族医药学会国际交流与合作分会常务副会长兼秘书长

（六）主编

杨　明　中国江西中医药大学副校长、教授、博士生导师，中药制剂
　　　　学家

卜海兵　中国原第309医院副院长、教授、高级工程师，医院管理、健
　　　　康科技专家

朱晓新　中国中医科学院中药研究所原书记、副所长、教授、博士生
　　　　导师，中药药理学家

（七）副主编

李　浩　中国武汉金银潭医院国家医疗队中医医疗组组长，中国中医
　　　　科学院西苑医院副院长、教授

林明贵　中国清华大学附属北京清华长庚医院新冠疫情专家组组长、
　　　　感染科主任、教授，中央保健委专家

刘良徛　中国江西中医药大学附属医院副院长、教授、博士生导师，
　　　　江西省新冠肺炎中医药防治专家组组长

（八）编委

周步高　中国江西中医药大学教授

张元兵　中国江西中医药大学教授、主任中医师

兰智慧　中国江西中医药大学教授、主任中医师

宋民宪　中国江西中医药大学教授

李守章　中国瑞典中医治疗中心、中国山东青岛市中西医结合医院、华
　　　　瑞和润中医机构副主任医师

秦承伟　中国援坦桑尼亚医疗队队长、山东省滨州医学院附属医院主任
　　　　医师

贾青良　尼泊尔中华医院院长

朱　明　中国湖南中方国际红十字医院院长

张　嵘　中国北京大学副教授

张磊昌　中国江西中医药大学副教授、副主任中医师

丁兆辉　中国江西中医药大学讲师、主治中医师

李明頔　澳大利亚 AHPRA 注册中医师，墨尔本皇家理工大学辅助医学

　　　　博士（在读）

（九）英文翻译

李涛安　中国江西中医药大学人文学院

余亚薇　中国江西中医药大学人文学院

任俊伟　中国江西中医药大学人文学院

涂宇明　中国江西中医药大学人文学院

郑鸿翔　中国江西中医药大学人文学院

杨具荣　中国江西中医药大学人文学院

谌志远　中国江西中医药大学人文学院

面向国际的中西医结合防治

新型冠状病毒肺炎

诊疗建议方案

一、临床表现特点

基于目前的流行病学调查，潜伏期一般为1~14天，多为3~7天。

以发热、干咳、乏力为主要表现。少数患者伴有恶寒、鼻塞、流涕、头痛、咽痛、肌痛、关节酸痛、食量减少、口干、口黏、无汗、腹泻、大便干燥等症状。重型病例多在发病一周后出现呼吸困难和/或低氧血症，严重者快速进展为急性呼吸窘迫综合征、脓毒症休克、难以纠正的代谢性酸中毒和出凝血功能障碍。值得注意的是重型、危重型患者病程中可为中低热，甚至无明显发热。

部分患者仅表现为低热、轻微乏力等，无肺炎表现，多在1周后恢复，但仍具传染性。

多数患者预后良好，少数患者病情转重或危重。老年人和有慢性基础疾病者预后较差，儿童病例症状相对较轻。

二、辅助检查

（一）一般检查

发病早期外周血白细胞总数正常或减少，可见淋巴细胞计数减少，部分患者可出现转氨酶、乳酸脱氢酶（LDH）、肌酶和肌红蛋白增高；部分危重者可见肌钙蛋白增高。多数患者C反应蛋白（CRP）和血沉升高，降钙素原正常。严重者D-二聚体升高，外周血淋巴细胞进行性减少。重型、危重型患者常有炎症因子升高。

（二）病原学及血清学检查

1. 病原学检查：采用RT-PCR和/或NGS方法在鼻咽拭子，痰和其他下呼吸道分泌物、血液、粪便等标本中可检测出新型冠状病毒核酸。检测下呼吸道标本（痰或气道抽取物）更加准确。标本采集后尽快送检。

2. 血清学检查：新型冠状病毒特异性IgM抗体多在发病3~5天后开始出现阳性，IgG抗体滴度恢复期较急性期有4倍及以上增高。

（三）胸部影像学

早期呈现多发小斑片影及间质改变，以肺外带明显。进而发展为双肺多发磨玻璃影、浸润影，严重者可出现肺实变，胸腔积液少见。

三、诊断标准

（一）疑似病例

结合下述流行病学史和临床表现综合分析：

1. 流行病学史

（1）发病前14天内有疫区及周边地区，或其他有病例报告社区的旅行史或居住史；

（2）发病前14天内与新型冠状病毒感染者有接触史；

（3）发病前14天内曾接触过来自疫区，或来自有病例报告社区的发热或有呼吸道症状的患者；

（4）聚集性发病（2周内在小范围如家庭、办公室、学校班级等场所，出现2例及以上发热和/或呼吸道症状的病例）。

2. 临床表现

（1）发热和/或呼吸道症状；

（2）具有上述新型冠状病毒性肺炎影像学特征；

（3）发病早期白细胞总数正常或降低，淋巴细胞计数正常或减少。

有流行病学史中的任何一条，且符合临床表现中任意2条。无明确流行病学史的，符合临床表现中的3条。

（二）确诊病例

疑似病例同时具备以下病原学或血清学证据之一者：

1. 实时荧光 RT-PCR 检测新型冠状病毒核酸阳性；

2. 病毒基因测序，与已知的新型冠状病毒高度同源；

3. 血清新型冠状病毒特异性 IgM 抗体和 IgG 抗体阳性；血清新型冠状病毒特异性 IgG 抗体由阴性转为阳性或恢复期较急性期 4 倍及以上升高。

四、鉴别诊断

（一）新型冠状病毒感染轻型表现需与其他病毒引起的上呼吸道感染相鉴别。

（二）新型冠状病毒性肺炎主要与流行性感冒病毒、腺病毒、呼吸道合胞病毒等其他已知病毒性肺炎及肺炎支原体感染鉴别，尤其是对疑似病例要尽可能采取包括快速抗原检测和多重 PCR 核酸检测等方法，对常见呼吸道病原体进行检测。

（三）还要与非感染性疾病，如血管炎、皮肌炎和机化性肺炎等鉴别。

五、预防干预建议

适用人群：普通人群中免疫力不足者、年老体弱者。

注意事项：孕妇禁用，使用过程中如有任何不适及时停用（见表 1）。

表1. 预防用药表

主方	兼症	加用方
匡扶正气散（附录1-1）袋泡剂（20目），5g/袋，用法：一次1袋，一天2次，开水冲服或用250ml水煎煮5分钟后饮用，服用一周即可。或玉屏风口服液（附录1-2）	若兼胃肠不适	藿香正气水（附录1-3）、藿香正气丸（附录1-4、1-5、1-6）
	若兼发热乏力	小柴胡颗粒（附录1-7）、清热八味胶囊（附录1-8）或连花清瘟胶囊（颗粒）（附录1-9、1-10）或金花清感颗粒（附录1-11）
	若兼全身酸痛	九味羌活丸（附录1-12）或川芎茶调颗粒（附录1-13）
	若兼咳嗽	通宣理肺丸（附录1-14、1-15）
	若兼胸闷	桂龙咳喘宁片（附录1-16）
	若兼咳嗽痰黄	鲜竹沥口服液（附录1-17）
	若兼咽痛咽干	银翘解毒丸（附录1-18）
	若兼便秘	三黄片（附录1-19）
	若咽干舌燥口渴	百合固金丸（附录1-20、1-21）
	若兼失眠	安神补心六味丸（附录1-22）

推荐针灸、电针、经皮穴位电刺激疗法，常规提高免疫力。

选穴：足三里（双侧），气海，中脘，如使用毫针，每次留针25~30分钟，针刺补法。如使用电针或经皮穴位电刺激疗法选择低频2Hz，电流强度10~20mA，隔日一次，每次15~20分钟。

六、分证与治疗

（一）疑似病例的防治（见表2）

表2. 疑似病例防治用药表

主方	兼症	加用方
玉屏风口服液（附录1-2）	若兼胃肠不适，舌质淡伴齿痕或淡红，苔白厚腐腻或白腻	藿香正气水（附录1-3）、藿香正气丸（附录1-4、1-5、1-6）
	若兼发热乏力，舌质淡或淡红，苔白腻	小柴胡颗粒（附录1-7）、清热八味胶囊（附录1-8）
	若兼全身酸痛，舌质淡或淡红，苔白腻	九味羌活丸（附录1-12）或川芎茶调颗粒（附录1-13）
	若兼咳嗽，舌质淡或淡红，苔白厚腻或白腻	通宣理肺丸（附录1-14、1-15）
	若兼胸闷，舌质淡或淡红，苔白厚腻或白腻	桂龙咳喘宁片（附录1-16）
	若兼咳嗽痰黄，舌质红，苔黄腻	鲜竹沥口服液（附录1-17）
	若兼咽痛咽干，舌质红，苔薄黄	银翘解毒丸（附录1-18）
	若兼便秘，舌质红，苔黄厚	三黄片（附录1-19）
	若咽干舌燥口渴，舌干少津	百合固金丸（附录1-20、1-21）
	若兼失眠，舌淡红，苔薄白	安神补心六味丸（附录1-22）

（二）轻型与普通型（疑似病例可参照轻型和普通治疗方案执行）

1. 中医辨证施治

（1）寒湿证（见表3）

临床表现：见低热（37.3℃≤T≤38.0℃），乏力，周身酸痛，咳嗽，咯痰，胸紧憋气，食欲差，恶心，呕吐，大便黏腻不爽。舌质淡伴齿痕或淡红，苔白厚腐腻或白腻，脉濡或滑。

表3. 轻型与普通型寒湿证用药表

主方	兼症	加用方
藿香正气（丸、水）（附录1-3、1-4、1-5、1-6）	若兼发热	小柴胡颗粒（附录1-7）
	若兼全身酸痛	九味羌活丸（附录1-12）或川芎茶调颗粒（附录1-13）
	若兼咳嗽	通宣理肺丸（附录1-14、1-15）
	若兼胸闷	桂龙咳喘宁片（附录1-16）

（2）湿热证（见表4）

临床表现：见低热（37.3℃≤T≤38.0℃）或不发热，微恶寒，乏力，头身困重，肌肉酸痛，干咳痰少，咽痛，口干不欲多饮，或伴有胸闷、呼吸困难，腹部胀满，无汗或汗出不畅，或见食欲差，恶心，呕吐，轻度腹泻或大便黏滞不爽。舌淡红，苔白厚腻或薄黄，脉滑数或濡。

表4. 轻型与普通型湿热证用药表

主方	兼症	加用方
清热八味胶囊（附录1-8）	若兼咳嗽痰黄	鲜竹沥口服液（附录1-17）
	若兼咽痛咽干	银翘解毒丸（附录1-18）
	若兼便秘	三黄片（附录1-19）
	若兼失眠焦虑	安神补心六味丸（附录1-22）

（3）针对以上疑似病例、轻型和普通型患者，推荐治疗方：

1）解毒益气散（附录1-23）

袋泡剂（粒径20目），5g/袋，用法：一次3袋，一天3次，开水冲服或用250ml水煎煮5分钟后饮用，一疗程3天。

2）清肺排毒汤

3）化湿败毒颗粒（附录1-24）

4）针灸、电针、经皮穴位电刺激疗法

选穴：合谷（双侧），足三里（双侧），太冲（双侧），神阙，如使用毫针，每次留针25~30分钟，平补平泻。如使用电针或经皮穴位电刺激疗法选择低频2Hz，电流强度10~20mA，每日一次，每次15~20分钟。

2. 基础治疗

（1）卧床休息，加强支持治疗，保证充分热量；注意水、电解质平衡，维持内环境稳定；密切监测生命体征、指氧饱和度等。

（2）根据病情监测血常规、尿常规、CRP、生化指标（转氨酶、心肌酶、肾功能等）、凝血功能、动脉血气分析、胸部影像学等。

（3）有胸闷喘息症状者及低氧血症者及时给予有效氧疗措施，包括鼻导管、面罩给氧和经鼻高流量氧疗。

3. 抗病毒治疗

目前尚无特别有效的新冠治疗药物，可试用α-干扰素（成人每次

500万U或相当剂量，加入灭菌注射用水2ml，每日2次雾化吸入）、利巴韦林（成人500mg/次，每日2至3次静脉输注，疗程不超过10天）、磷酸氯喹（18~65岁成人。体重大于50kg者，每次500mg、每日2次，疗程7天；体重小于50kg者，第一、二天每次500mg，每日2次，第三至第七天每次500mg、每日1次）。

要注意上述药物的不良反应、禁忌证（如患有心脏疾病者禁用氯喹）以及与其他药物联合应用等问题。上述药物均需在临床应用中进一步评价其疗效。不建议同时应用3种及以上抗病毒药物，出现不可耐受的毒副作用时应停止使用相关药物并对症处理。

4. 抗菌药物治疗

避免盲目或不恰当使用抗菌药物，尤其是联合使用广谱抗菌药物。WBC>1万以上和/或N>85%考虑使用，抗生素使用一般5~7d。结合临床选用抗生素种类。

（三）重型

1. 重型、危重型临床预警指标

（1）成人

①外周血淋巴细胞进行性下降；

②外周血炎症因子如IL-6、C反应蛋白进行性上升；

③乳酸进行性升高；

④肺内病变在短期内迅速进展。

（2）儿童

①呼吸频率增快；

②精神反应差、嗜睡；

③乳酸进行性升高；

④影像学显示双侧或多肺叶浸润、胸腔积液或短期内病变快速进展；

⑤月龄以下的婴儿或有基础疾病（先天性心脏病、支气管肺发育不良、

呼吸道畸形、异常血红蛋白、重度营养不良等），有免疫缺陷或低下（长期使用免疫抑制剂）。

2. 中医辨证施治

（1）疫毒闭肺证

临床表现：发热面红（38.0℃<T≤39.0℃），咳嗽，痰黄黏少，或痰中带血，喘憋气促（RR>30次/min；或静息状态下，指氧饱和度≤93%；或动脉血氧分压（PaO$_2$）/吸氧浓度（FiO$_2$）≤300mmHg；或肺部影像学显示24~48小时内病灶明显进展>50%者），疲乏倦怠，口干苦黏，恶心不食，大便不畅，小便短赤。舌红，苔黄腻，脉滑数。

推荐中成药：牛黄清心丸（附录1-25）或清热八味胶囊。

（2）气营两燔证（见表5）

临床表现：高热心烦口渴（T>39.0℃），喘憋气促（喘憋气促（RR>30次/min；或静息状态下，指氧饱和度≤93%；或动脉血氧分压（PaO$_2$）/吸氧浓度（FiO$_2$）≤300mmHg；肺部影像学显示24~48小时内病灶明显进展>50%者），神志昏迷，或皮下出血或吐血、或四肢抽搐。舌绛少苔或无苔，脉沉细数，或浮大而数。

表5. 重型气营两燔证用药表

主方	兼症	加用方
安宫牛黄丸（附录1-26）合用片仔癀（附录1-27）	若兼咳嗽	通宣理肺丸（附录1-14、1-15）
	若喘促、出汗	生脉饮口服液（附录1-28）
	若痰多色黄	鲜竹沥口服液（附录1-17）
	若咯血	云南白药（附录1-29）

3. 基础治疗

（1）氧疗；

（2）老年弱者，可考虑丙种球蛋白支持治疗3~5d；

（3）根据生化指标适当选择营养支持疗法。

4. 中药注射剂

（1）指征：发热（低热或高热）。5%GS或0.9%NS100~250ml+喜炎平注射液（附录1-30）50~100ml静脉滴注，一日2次。

（2）指征：有痰色黄，或发热。5%GS或0.9%NS100~250ml+痰热清注射液（附录1-31）20~40ml，静脉滴注，一日1次。

（3）指征：高热，神志不清。5%GS或0.9%NS100~250ml+醒脑静注射液（附录1-32）20~40ml，静脉滴注，一日1次。

（4）指征：肺影像呈现新冠肺炎特征。0.9%NS100+血必净注射液（附录1-33）50ml，静脉滴注，一日2次。可考虑与上述注射剂联合使用。

（5）指征：存在免疫抑制情况。0.9%氯化钠注射液250ml加参麦注射液（附录1-34）100ml，一日2次。

（6）指征：出现休克。0.9%氯化钠注射液250ml加参附注射液（附录1-35）100ml，一日2次。

5. 对症治疗

（1）发热：≥38.5℃，可予柴胡注射液（附录1-36）（4ml/次，1~3次/d），或可予塞来昔布（0.2g/次，1~2次/d），或双氯芬酸钠栓（25mg~50mg/次，1~2次/d）。

（2）咳嗽：可予右美沙芬（15~30mg/次，3~4次/d），或惠菲宁（10ml/次，3~4次/d）。

（3）痰多难咯，予氨溴索（30mg/次，3~4次/d），或乙酰半胱氨酸泡腾片（0.6g/次，1~3次/d）。

（4）喘息伴肺部哮鸣音，予茶碱缓释片（1~2片/次，2次/d）。

（5）腹泻，可予蒙脱石散（附录1-37）（1~2袋/次，3次/d）。

6. 抗生素使用

指征：有细菌感染征象，如WBC>1.0万以上和/或中性>85%时考虑使用，抗生素使用一般5~7d。结合临床选用抗生素种类。

如：0.9%NS100ml+头孢哌酮/他唑巴坦3g静滴一日2~3次，和/或

0.9%NS100ml+莫西沙星0.4g 静滴一日1次；或0.9%NS100ml+美洛培南1.0g 静滴一日3次（每8小时1次）。

7. 抗病毒药使用

可试用α-干扰素雾化吸入（成人每次500万U，加入灭菌注射用水2ml，每日2次）；利巴韦林（成人500mg/次静滴，2~3次/d）；磷酸氯喹（成人500mg，2次/d）疗程均不超过10天。

8. 激素使用

原则上避免使用或慎用激素，即使使用也要遵循短期使用原则（3~5天），建议剂量不超过相当于甲泼尼龙1~2mg/（kg·d）。使用指征：呼吸困难明显、严重低氧血症，肺部影像进展明显，和/或炎症指标明显升高。

9. 儿童符合下列任何一条，可参照成人标准进行分型治疗

（1）出现气促(<2月龄,RR≥60次/min；2~12月龄,RR≥50次/min；1~5岁,RR≥40次/min；>5岁，RR≥30次/min)，除外发热和哭闹的影响；

（2）静息状态下，指氧饱和度≤92%；

（3）辅助呼吸（呻吟、鼻翼翕动、三凹征），发绀，间歇性呼吸暂停；

（4）出现嗜睡、惊厥；

（5）拒食或喂养困难，有脱水征。

（四）危重型

临床表现：呼吸困难、动辄气喘（需要机械通气），伴神志异常（出现休克或合并其他器官功能衰竭需ICU监护治疗），烦躁，汗出肢冷。舌质紫暗，苔厚腻或燥，脉浮大无根。

1. 治疗原则：在对症治疗的基础上，积极防治并发症，治疗基础疾病，预防继发感染，及时进行器官功能支持。

2. 中医辨证施治

内闭外脱证（见表6）

临床表现：呼吸困难，动辄气喘或需要机械通气，伴神志昏迷,烦躁，汗出肢冷。舌质紫暗，苔厚腻或燥，脉浮大无根。

表6. 危重型内闭外脱证用药表

主方	兼症	加用方
生脉饮口服液（附录1-28）	昏迷兼面红、身热、苔黄、脉数者	安宫牛黄丸（伴高热首选）（附录1-26）
	昏迷兼面青、身凉、苔白、脉迟者	苏合香丸（附录1-38）

3. 中药注射剂、抗生素使用、激素使用：同重型。

4. 呼吸支持

（1）氧疗：重型患者应当接受鼻导管或面罩吸氧，并及时评估呼吸窘迫和/或低氧血症是否缓解。

（2）高流量鼻导管氧疗或无创机械通气：当患者接受标准氧疗后呼吸窘迫和/或低氧血症无法缓解时，可考虑使用高流量鼻导管氧疗或无创通气。若短时间（1~2小时）内病情无改善甚至恶化，应当及时进行气管插管和有创机械通气。

（3）有创机械通气：采用肺保护性通气策略，即小潮气量（6~8ml/kg理想体重）和低水平气道平台压力（≤30cmH$_2$O）进行机械通气，以减少呼吸机相关肺损伤。在保证气道平台压≤35cmH$_2$O时，可适当采用高PEEP，保持气道温化湿化，避免长时间镇静，早期唤醒患者并进行肺康复治疗。较多患者存在人机不同步，应当及时使用镇静以及肌松剂。根据气道分泌物情况，选择密闭式吸痰，必要时行支气管镜检查采取相应治疗。

（4）挽救治疗：对于严重ARDS患者，建议进行肺复张。在人力资源充足的情况下，每天应当进行12小时以上的俯卧位通气。俯卧位机械通气效果不佳者，如条件允许，应当尽快考虑体外膜氧合器（ECMO）。其相关指征：①在FiO$_2$>90%时，氧合指数小于80mmHg，持续3~4小时以上；②气道平台压≥35cmH$_2$O。单纯呼吸衰竭患者，首选VV-ECMO模式；若需要循环支持，则选用VA-ECMO模式。在基础疾病得以控制，心肺功能有恢复迹象时，可开始撤机试验。

5. 循环支持

在充分液体复苏的基础上，改善微循环，使用血管活性药物，密切监测患者血压、心率和尿量的变化，以及动脉血气分析中乳酸和碱剩余，必要时进行无创或有创血流动力学监测，如超声多普勒法、超声心动图、有创血压或持续心排血量（PiCCO）监测。在救治过程中，注意液体平衡策略，避免过量和不足。如果发现患者心率突发增加大于基础值的20%或血压下降大约基础值20%以上时，若伴有皮肤灌注不良和尿量减少等表现时，应密切观察患者是否存在脓毒症休克、消化道出血或心功能衰竭等情况。

6. 肾衰竭和肾替代治疗

危重症患者的肾功能损伤应积极寻找导致肾功能损伤的原因，如低灌注和药物等因素。对于肾衰竭患者的治疗应注重体液平衡、酸碱平衡和电解质平衡，在营养支持治疗方面应注意氮平衡、热量和微量元素等补充。重症患者可选择连续性肾替代治疗（continuous renal replacement therapy, CRRT）。其指征包括：（1）高钾血症；（2）酸中毒；（3）肺水肿或水负荷过重；（4）多器官功能不全时的液体管理。

7. 血液净化治疗

血液净化系统包括血浆置换、吸附、灌流、血液/血浆滤过等，能清除炎症因子，阻断"细胞因子风暴"，从而减轻炎症反应对机体的损伤，可用于重型、危重型患者细胞因子风暴早中期的救治。

8. 免疫治疗

对于双肺广泛病变者及重型患者，且实验室检测IL-6水平升高者，可试用托珠单抗治疗。首次剂量4~8mg/kg，推荐剂量为400mg、0.9%生理盐水稀释至100ml，输注时间大于1小时；首次用药疗效不佳者，可在12小时后追加应用一次（剂量同前），累计给药次数最多为2次，单次最大剂量不超过

800mg。注意过敏反应，有结核等活动性感染者禁用。

9. 其他治疗措施

对于氧合指标进行性恶化、影像学进展迅速、机体炎症反应过度激活状态的患者，酌情短期内（3~5日）使用糖皮质激素，建议剂量不超过相当于甲泼尼龙1~2ml/（kg·d），应当注意较大剂量糖皮质激素由于免疫抑制作用，会延缓对冠状病毒的清除；可静脉给予血必净注射液100ml/次，每日2次治疗；可使用肠道微生态调节剂，维持肠道微生态平衡。

儿童重型、危重型病例可酌情考虑给予静脉滴注丙种球蛋白。患有重型或危重型新型冠状病毒性肺炎的孕妇应积极终止妊娠，剖宫产为首选。

患者常存在焦虑恐惧情绪，应当加强心理疏导。

七、恢复期

（一）中医辨证施治

1. 肺脾气虚证（见表7）

临床表现：气短，疲倦乏力，食欲差，恶心，呕吐，腹胀，大便无力，轻度腹泻或大便黏滞不爽。舌淡胖，苔白腻。

表7. 恢复期肺脾气虚证用药表

主方	兼症	加用方
参苓白术散（附录1-39），或参苓白术丸（附录1-40），或补中益气丸（附录1-41），或香砂六君丸（附录1-42）	抑郁、精神紧张者	逍遥丸（附录1-43）

2. 气阴两虚证（见表8）

临床表现：乏力，气短，口干，口黏，心悸，汗多，低热或不热，干咳少痰。舌干少津，脉细或虚无力。

表8. 恢复期气阴两虚证用药表

主方	兼症	加用方
生脉饮口服液（附录1-28） 或百合固金丸（附录1-21）	食欲差者	健胃消食片（附录1-45）

3. 痰凝血瘀证（见表9）

临床表现：胸闷气憋，活动后呼吸困难，阵发性干咳、呛咳为主，或咳少量白痰。舌质淡暗，苔薄白或腻，脉沉弦或涩。

胸部CT提示肺间质病变征象明显。

表9. 恢复期痰凝血瘀证用药表

主方	兼症	加用方
桂枝茯苓丸（附录1-44），或温肺化纤颗粒	食欲差者	健胃消食片（附录1-45）
	活动后呼吸困难，精神疲惫，不欲言语等气虚突出者	补中益气丸或散（附录1-41）
	口干，咽燥，苔少等阴虚者	生脉饮口服液（附录1-28）
	咳嗽明显者	通宣理肺丸（附录1-14、1-15）

（二）中医适宜技术使用

1. 针灸疗法

操作方法及频次：毫针每日或每隔日一次，每次留针25~30分钟，行针刺补法。如给予电针或经皮穴位电刺激，给予2Hz，10~20mA电刺激，每日或隔日一次，每次15~20分钟。如穴位艾灸刺激，则早晚各一次，每次15~20分钟。

【基础选穴】大椎，足三里，肺俞，膈俞。

（1）肺脾气虚证

【选穴】太渊、膻中、气海、关元。痰多者加丰隆、太白；畏寒者加风门艾灸；腹胀便溏加天枢。

（2）肺胃阴虚证

【选穴】太渊、膏肓、太溪、三阴交。咯血加孔最；腹胀加中脘，便秘加天枢。

（3）余邪未尽，气阴两伤证

【选穴】肾俞、鱼际、太渊、太溪、三阴交。喘甚者加定喘；失眠加内关、神门。

2. 耳针疗法

【选穴】肺、平喘、神门、大肠、内分泌等。

【贴敷法】可选中药王不留行籽取穴贴敷，每日用手指轻压1~2分钟，每三天更换。

【禁忌】皮肤破溃或皮肤过敏、瘢痕体质患者禁用。

3. 穴位贴

可选白芥子、细辛、川芎、苍术等研磨成细粉，制作成药饼进行贴敷。

【选穴】肺俞、定喘、膏肓、膻中、丰隆等。

【频次】每日一次，每次4~6个小时。

【禁忌】孕妇、咯血、皮肤破溃或皮肤过敏、瘢痕体质患者禁用。

4. 艾灸

用艾条，采用循经往返灸，从风门到膈俞，距皮肤1.5~3cm左右。操作时间约20分钟，隔日一次。

八、解除隔离和出院后注意事项

（一）出院标准

1. 体温恢复正常3天以上；

2. 呼吸道症状明显好转；

3. 肺部影像学显示急性渗出性病变明显改善；

4. 连续两次痰、鼻咽拭子等呼吸道标本核酸检测阴性（采样时间至少间隔24小时）。

满足以上条件者可出院。

（二）出院后注意事项

1. 定点医院要做好与患者居住地基层医疗机构间的联系，共享病历资料，及时将出院患者信息推送至患者辖区或居住地居委会和基层医疗卫生机构。

2. 患者出院后，建议应继续进行14天的隔离管理和健康状况监测，佩戴口罩，有条件的居住在通风良好的单人房间，减少与家人的近距离密切接触，分餐饮食，做好手卫生，避免外出活动。

3. 建议在出院后第2周和第4周到医院随访、复诊。

附录 1

处方、成方制剂标准基本信息

■ 1. 匡扶正气散

【处方来源】由中国国家级名老中医、北京中医药大学刘景源教授选用（公元1127—1279年）金·张元素《医学启源》记载的《生脉散》、元代（公元1347年）《丹溪心法》记载的《玉屏风散》、宋代陈师文等撰《太平惠民和剂局方》记载的《藿香正气散》合方加减化裁而成。

【组成】广藿香、紫苏叶、白芷、麦冬、防风、黄芪、党参、五味子、白术、北沙参、石斛、甜叶菊。

【功能】气阴双补，增强免疫力，用于未感人群预防使用。

■ 2. 玉屏风口服液

【处方来源】原玉屏风散，出自元代（公元1347年）《丹溪心法》。

【标准来源】《中国药典》2020年版一部第781页。

【组成】黄芪、防风、麸炒白术。

【功能】益气，固表，止汗。

■ **3. 藿香正气水**

【处方来源】 陈师文等撰《太平惠民和剂局方》，宋代（公元1151年）。

【标准来源】《中国药典》2020年版一部第1881页。

【组成】 苍术、陈皮、厚朴（姜制）、白芷、茯苓、大腹皮、生半夏、甘草浸膏、广藿香油、紫苏叶油。

【功能】 解表化湿，理气和中。

■ **4. 藿香正气丸（大蜜丸）**

【处方来源】 陈师文等撰《太平惠民和剂局方》，宋代（公元1151年）。

【标准来源】 中国国家中成药标准汇编内科肺系（一）分册第455页。

【组成】 苍术、陈皮、厚朴（姜制）、白芷、茯苓、大腹皮、半夏（姜制）、甘草、广藿香、紫苏叶。

【功能】 解表退热，和中理气。

5. 藿香正气丸（水蜜丸）

【处方来源】 陈师文等撰《太平惠民和剂局方》，宋代
（公元1151年）。

【标准来源】 中国国家中成药标准汇编内科肺系（一）
分册第455页。

【组成】 苍术、陈皮、厚朴（姜制）、白芷、茯苓、
大腹皮、半夏（姜制）、甘草、广藿香、
紫苏叶。

【功能】 解表退热，和中理气。

6. 藿香正气丸（水丸）

【处方来源】 原方出自（公元1151年）宋·陈师文等撰
《太平惠民和剂局方》。

【标准来源】 中国国家中成药标准汇编内科肺系（一）
分册第455页。

【组成】 苍术、陈皮、厚朴（姜制）、白芷、茯苓、
大腹皮、半夏（姜制）、甘草、广藿香、
紫苏叶。

【功能】 解表退热，和中理气。

7. 小柴胡颗粒

【处方来源】 《伤寒杂病论》，汉代（公元219年）。

【标准来源】 《中国药典》2020年版一部第605页。

【组成】 柴胡、黄芩、姜半夏、党参、生姜、甘草、大枣。

【功能】 解表散热，疏肝和胃。

8. 清热八味胶囊

【处方来源】 出自公元8世纪的《四部医典》，是传统蒙药方剂，亦称蒙药八尊。

【标准来源】 中国国家食品药品监督管理总局国家药品标准ZZ-8404-1。

【组成】 檀香、石膏、红花、苦地丁、瞿麦、胡黄连、麦冬、人工牛黄。

【功能】 清热解毒。用于脏腑热，肺热咳嗽，痰中带血，肝火肋痛。

9. 连花清瘟胶囊

【处方来源】 连花清瘟同"莲花清瘟"组方来源于治疗热性病流行的著名方剂（公元1798年）清·吴瑭（鞠通）著《温病条辨》中的银翘散和（公元219年）汉·张机（仲景）著《伤寒论》中的麻杏石甘汤，由两方化裁制成。

【标准来源】《中国药典》2020年版一部第1014页。

【组成】 连翘、金银花、炙麻黄、炒苦杏仁、石膏、板蓝根、绵马贯众、鱼腥草、广藿香、大黄、红景天、薄荷脑、甘草。

【功能】 清瘟解毒，宣肺泄热。

10. 连花清瘟颗粒

【处方来源】 连花清瘟同"莲花清瘟"组方来源于治疗热性病流行的著名方剂（公元1798年）清·吴瑭（鞠通）著《温病条辨》中的银翘散和（公元219年）汉·张机（仲景）著《伤寒论》中的麻杏石甘汤，由两方化裁制成。

【标准来源】《中国药典》2020年版一部第1015页。

【组成】 连翘、金银花、炙麻黄、炒苦杏仁、石膏、板蓝根、绵马贯众、鱼腥草、广藿香、大黄、红景天、薄荷脑、甘草。

【功能】 清瘟解毒，宣肺泄热。

■ 11. 金花清感颗粒

【处方来源】 原方金花清感方参考（公元219年）汉·张机（仲景）著《伤寒论》，（公元1641年）明·吴又可著《瘟疫论》，（公元1798年）清·吴瑭（鞠通）著《温病条辨》等中医经典古籍中的百余个处方，借鉴临床专家成果，历经反复筛选并优化而成。

【标准来源】 中国国家药监局标准YBZ00392016。

【组成】 金银花、石膏、蜜麻黄、炒苦杏仁、黄芩、连翘、浙贝母、知母、牛蒡子、青蒿、薄荷、甘草。

【功能】 疏风宣肺，清热解毒。

■ 12. 九味羌活丸

【处方来源】 原方九味羌活方出自金代名医张元素，后来元代医家王好古师从张元素之徒李杲，首次将九味羌活汤录于《此事难知》中（公元1279—1368年）。

【标准来源】 《中国药典》2020年版一部第501页。

【组成】 羌活、防风、苍术、细辛、川芎、白芷、黄芩、甘草、地黄。

【功能】 疏风解表，散寒除湿。

13. 川芎茶调颗粒

【处方来源】 川芎茶调颗粒源于宋代《太平惠民和剂局方》的川芎茶调散（公元1078—1085年）。

【标准来源】《中国药典》2020年版一部第546页。

【组成】 川芎、白芷、羌活、细辛、防风、荆芥、薄荷、甘草。

【功能】 疏风止痛。

14. 通宣理肺丸（大蜜丸）

【处方来源】 出自明代王肯堂《证治准绳》，原为明代古方"紫苏饮"加减（公元1602年）。

【标准来源】《中国药典》2020年版一部第1571页。

【组成】 紫苏叶、前胡、桔梗、苦杏仁、麻黄、甘草、陈皮、半夏（制）、茯苓、枳壳（炒）、黄芩。

【功能】 解表散寒，宣肺止咳。

■ **15. 通宣理肺丸（水蜜丸）**

【处方来源】 出自明代王肯堂《证治准绳》，原为明代古方"紫苏饮"加减（公元 1602 年）。

【标准来源】《中国药典》2020 年版一部第 1571 页。

【组成】 紫苏叶、前胡、桔梗、苦杏仁、麻黄、甘草、陈皮、半夏（制）、茯苓、枳壳（炒）、黄芩。

【功能】 解表散寒，宣肺止咳。

■ **16. 桂龙咳喘宁片**

【处方来源】 东汉张仲景所著《金匮要略》（公元 206 年）。

【标准来源】《中国药典》2020 年版一部第 1431 页。

【组成】 桂枝、龙骨、白芍、生姜、大枣、炙甘草、牡蛎、黄连、法半夏、瓜蒌皮、炒苦杏仁。

【功能】 止咳化痰，降气平喘。

■ **17. 鲜竹沥口服液**

【处方来源】《本草经集注》，约公元480—498年。

【标准来源】 中国卫生部药品标准中药材第一册（1992
年版）第99页、国家药监局单页标准
（2004）。

【组成】 禾木科植物粉绿竹Phyllostachys glauca
McClure、净竹Phyllostachysnuda McClure
及同属数种植物的鲜杆经加热后自然沥
出的液体。

【功能】 清热化痰。

■ **18. 银翘解毒丸**

【处方来源】〔清〕《温病条辨》，公元1798年，清·吴
瑭（鞠通）著。

【标准来源】 中国卫生部药品标准中药成方制剂第
十九册第200页。

【组成】 金银花、连翘、薄荷、荆芥、淡豆豉、
牛蒡子（炒）、桔梗、淡竹叶、甘草。

【功能】 疏风解表，清热解毒。

19. 三黄片

【处方来源】 三黄片的处方源于东汉时期医圣张仲景所著《金匮要略》（公元206年）中"泻心汤"一方，历经千年而不衰。该方由大黄、黄芩、黄连三药组成，故名"三黄"。

【标准来源】《中国药典》2020年版一部第517页。

【组成】 大黄、盐酸小檗碱、黄芩浸膏。

【功能】 清热解毒，泻火通便。

20. 百合固金丸（浓缩丸）

【处方来源】 由百合固金丸浓缩而来。百合固金丸出自清代（公元1682年）汪昂《医方集解》。

【标准来源】 中国药典2020年版一部第880页。

【组成】 百合、地黄、熟地黄、麦冬、玄参、川贝母、当归、白芍、桔梗、甘草。

【功能】 养阴润肺，化痰止咳。

■ **21. 百合固金丸**

【处方来源】 清代（1682年）汪昂《医方集解》。

【标准来源】《中国药典》2020年版一部第879页。

【组成】 百合、地黄、熟地黄、麦冬、玄参、川
贝母、当归、白芍、桔梗、甘草。

【功能】 养阴润肺，化痰止咳。

■ **22. 安神补心六味丸**

【处方来源】 出自8世纪宇妥·宁玛云丹贡布所著《四
部医典》。

【标准来源】 中国国家食品药品监督管理总局国家药
品标准ZZ-8324-1。

【组成】 牛心、木香、枫香脂、丁香、肉豆蔻、
广枣。

【功能】 祛"赫依"，镇静，用于心慌、气短。

■ 23. 解毒益气散

【处方来源】 由中国国家级名老中医、北京中医药大
学刘景源教授选用经典古方《止嗽散》
元代（公元1347年）《丹溪心法》记载的
《玉屏风散》，宋代陈师文等撰《太平惠
民和剂局方》记载的《藿香正气散》合
方加减化裁而成。

【组成】 广藿香、紫苏叶、白芷、党参、清半夏、
黄芪、北沙参、麦冬、防风、浙贝母、
金银花、黄芩、薤白、杏仁、瓜蒌皮、
炙款冬花、炙紫菀、桑白皮、桑叶、石
斛、甜叶菊。

【功能】 药物寒温并用、祛邪扶正并用。补气与
补阴并用，药性平和。适用于疑似病例、
轻型、普通型患者，重症患者配合西医
支持疗法使用。

24. 化湿败毒颗粒

【处方来源】 中国国家卫健委印发新型冠状病毒肺炎诊疗方案（试行第七版）。

【组成】 麻黄、杏仁、石膏、甘草、广藿香、厚朴、苍术、草果、法半夏、茯苓、赤芍、大黄、黄芪、葶苈子。

【功能】 化湿辟秽，宣肺通腑，活血解毒。

25. 牛黄清心丸

【处方来源】 陈师文等撰《太平惠民和剂局方》，宋代（公元1151年）。

【标准来源】《中国药典》2020年版一部第690页。

【组成】 牛黄、当归、川芎、甘草、山药、黄芩、炒苦杏仁、大豆黄卷、大枣、白术（炒）、茯苓、桔梗、防风、柴胡、阿胶、干姜、白芍、人参、六神曲（炒）、肉桂、麦冬、白蔹、蒲黄（炒）、人工麝香、冰片、水牛角浓缩粉、羚羊角、朱砂、雄黄。

【功能】 清热解毒，开窍安神。

26. 安宫牛黄丸

【处方来源】 清·吴鞠通《温病条辨》上焦篇第16条。

【标准来源】《中国药典》2020年版一部第930页、勘误、增补本第95页。

【组成】 牛黄、水牛角浓缩粉、人工麝香、珍珠、朱砂、雄黄、黄连、黄芩、栀子、郁金、冰片。

【功能】 清热解毒，镇惊开窍。

27. 片仔癀

【处方来源】 该药原是明朝太医的秘方，明朝动乱中，档案尽皆流失，包括明时太医的秘方都不见经传。唯独可在李时珍的《本草纲目》中对三七的记载中获知一二，书中记载三七产于南方深山，既稀又贵，用三七入药传入宫廷，再配置成方，用特殊工艺制作成片仔癀，后定为宫廷秘方。1956年纳入漳州制药厂。

【标准来源】《中国药典》2020年版一部第703页。

【组成】 牛黄、麝香、三七、蛇胆等。

【功能】 清热解毒，凉血化瘀，消肿止痛。

28. 生脉饮口服液

【处方来源】 生脉饮为补益方剂之一，出自（公元 1127—1279年）金·张元素《医学启源》。

【标准来源】 中国卫生部药品标准中药成方制剂第 十二册第39页。

【组成】 党参、麦冬、五味子。

【功能】 益气复脉，养阴生津。

29. 云南白药

【处方来源】 云南白药原名"焕章百宝丹"，由曲焕章 于1902年炮制成功。

【标准来源】 《中国药典》2020年版一部第636页。

【组成】 三七、重楼等。

【功能】 清热解毒，镇惊开窍。

30. 喜炎平注射液

【处方来源】 《江西省药品标准》，1982年版。

【标准来源】 中国国家中成药标准汇编 内科肺系（二）
分册第455页、修订标准WS-10863（ZD-
0863）-2002-2011Z。

【组成】 穿心莲内酯磺化物。

【功能】 清热解毒，止咳止痢。

31. 痰热清注射液

【处方来源】 在双黄连的基础上加入清热类药材山羊
角和熊胆粉而成。双黄连依古方"大连
翘汤"和"银翘散"组方。大连翘汤
来源于《直指小儿》卷五：宋·杨士瀛
（仁斋）撰于景定元年（公元1260年）。
银翘散来源于《温病条辨》，公元1798
年，清·吴瑭（鞠通）著。

【标准来源】 新药转正标准75册第8页、中国国家药
监局标准YBZ00912003-2007Z-2009。

【组成】 黄芩、熊胆粉、山羊角、金银花、连翘。

【功能】 清热，化痰，解毒。

32. 醒脑静注射液

【处方来源】《中华人民共和国卫生部药品标准中药成方制剂第十七册》，现代（公元1998年）它是由祖国医学传统名方——安宫牛黄丸经减味而成，安宫牛黄丸方剂来源于《温病条辨》清代，公元1798年。

【标准来源】中国卫生部药品标准中药成方制剂第十七册第278页。

【组成】人工麝香、郁金、冰片、栀子。

【功能】清热解毒，凉血活血，开窍醒脑。

33. 血必净注射液

【处方来源】国家食品药品监督管理局标准颁布件，现代（公元2012年）。我国中西医结合急救医学奠基人王今达教授以古方血府逐瘀汤为基础精炼出的静脉制剂。血府逐瘀汤来源《医林改错》，初版于道光十年（公元1830年）。

【标准来源】中国YBZ01242004-2010Z-2012。

【组成】红花、赤芍、川芎、丹参、当归。

【功能】化瘀解毒。

■ **34. 参麦注射液**

【处方来源】由红参和麦冬两味药材制备而成的中药复方制剂。其成分源于明朝秦景明的《证因脉治》生脉饮，刊于1706年。

【标准来源】中国卫生部药品标准中药成方制剂第十八册第170页、标准修订件ZGB2010-7、标准修订件2011B011。

【组成】红参、麦冬。

【功能】益气固脱，养阴生津，生脉。

■ **35. 参附注射液**

【处方来源】处方来源于经典方剂"参附汤"。"参附汤"始见于（公元1253年）南宋·严用和《严氏济生方》。

【标准来源】中国中药部颁第18册 Z18-167 标准编号：WS3-B-3427-98。

【组成】红参、黑附片提取物，主要含人参皂苷、水溶性生物碱。

【功能】回阳救逆，益气固脱。

36. 柴胡注射液

【处方来源】 柴胡注射液是柴胡或狭叶柴胡经水蒸气蒸馏法制成的饱和水溶液,卫生部药品标准中药成方制剂第十七册。

【标准来源】 中国卫生部药品标准中药成方制剂第十七册第211页、国家中成药标准汇编内科肺系(一)分册第416页、SFDA标准颁布件(2011)。

【组成】 北柴胡。

【功能】 清热解表。

37. 蒙脱石散

【处方来源】 现代方剂,矿物药。

【标准来源】《中国药典》2020年版二部第1723页。

【组成】 蒙脱石。

【功能】 止泻。

38. 苏合香丸

【处方来源】 宋《太平惠民和剂局方》公元1151年。

【标准来源】《中国药典》2020年版一部 第996页。

【组成】 苏合香、安息香、冰片、水牛角浓缩粉、人工麝香、檀香、沉香、丁香、香附、木香、乳香（制）、荜茇、白术、诃子肉、朱砂。

【功能】 芳香开窍，行气止痛。

39. 参苓白术散

【处方来源】《太平惠民和剂局方》，公元1078—1085年。

【标准来源】 中国药典2020年版一部第1223页。

【组成】 人参、茯苓、白术（炒）、山药、白扁豆（炒）、莲子、薏苡仁（炒）、砂仁、桔梗、甘草。

【功能】 补脾胃，益肺气。

40. 参苓白术丸

【处方来源】 由参苓白术散发展而来,《太平惠民和剂局方》,公元1078—1085年。

【标准来源】《中国药典》2020年版一部第1222页。

【组成】 人参、茯苓、麸炒白术、山药、炒白扁豆、莲子、麸炒薏苡仁、砂仁、桔梗、甘草。

【功能】 补脾胃,益肺气。

41. 补中益气丸

【处方来源】 由补中益气汤转换剂型而得,补中益气汤,出自金代(公元1249年)李东垣所著的《脾胃论》。

【标准来源】《中国药典》2020年版一部第1063页。

【组成】 炙黄芪、党参、炙甘草、白术(炒)、当归、升麻、柴胡、陈皮、生姜、大枣。

【功能】 补中益气,升阳举陷。

■ 42. 香砂六君丸

【处方来源】 公元1682年,《医方集解》。

【标准来源】《中国药典》2020年版一部第1292页。

【组成】 木香、砂仁、党参、白术（炒）、茯苓、炙甘草、陈皮、半夏（姜制）。

【功能】 益气健脾，和胃。

■ 43. 逍遥丸

【处方来源】 逍遥丸是逍遥散由煮散剂演变为丸剂而成；逍遥散源自《太平惠民合剂局方》，公元1078—1085年。

【标准来源】《中国药典》2020年版一部第1461页。

【组成】 柴胡、当归、白芍、麸炒白术、茯苓、炙甘草、薄荷、生姜。

【功能】 疏肝健脾，养血调经。

44. 桂枝茯苓丸

【处方来源】 东汉张仲景所著《金匮要略》（公元206年）。

【标准来源】《中国药典》2020年版一部第1439页。

【组成】 桂枝、茯苓、牡丹皮、赤芍、桃仁。

【功能】 活血，化瘀，消癥。

45. 健胃消食片

【处方来源】 原方胃消食片，出自明代王肯堂《证治准绳》（公元1602年）。

【标准来源】《中国药典》2020年版一部第1474页。

【组成】 太子参、陈皮、山药、炒麦芽、山楂。

【功能】 健胃消食。

新冠肺炎临床证候评分量表

姓名（编号）：　　　　性别：　　　　年龄：　　　　联系方式：

入院日期：			总分：	
项目	无0	轻3	中6	重9
发热	□$_0$无	□$_3$37.3~38.5℃	□$_6$38.6~39.5℃	□$_9$39.5℃以上
恶寒	□$_0$无	□$_3$微恶风	□$_6$恶寒，加衣被不减	□$_9$寒战
头身痛	□$_0$无	□$_3$轻微头身痛，时做时止	□$_6$持续头身痛，但可忍	□$_9$头身剧痛，疼痛难忍
头身重	□$_0$无	□$_3$轻微头身重	□$_6$持续头身重，活动减少	□$_9$持续头身重，难以活动
乏力	□$_0$无	□$_3$乏力，不影响工作	□$_6$乏力，活动减少	□$_9$乏力，不欲动
汗出	□$_0$无	□$_3$偶有汗出	□$_6$少汗，未湿衣襟	□$_9$大汗淋漓
咳嗽	□$_0$无	□$_3$偶咳	□$_6$咳声阵作	□$_9$咳嗽连声频作
咳痰	□$_0$无	□$_3$时咳痰	□$_6$常咳痰	□$_9$常咳痰且量多
鼻塞	□$_0$无	□$_3$轻微	□$_6$通气不畅，流涕或黄涕	□$_9$持续不畅，流涕量多
咽痛	□$_0$无	□$_3$轻微	□$_6$干痛，吞咽时痛	□$_9$灼痛，吞咽剧痛
咽干	□$_0$无	□$_3$轻微	□$_6$咽干，偶欲饮水	□$_9$咽干，时欲饮水
气短	□$_0$无	□$_3$轻微	□$_6$气短明显，但不影响活动	□$_9$气短不能活动
喘促	□$_0$无	□$_3$喘促偶发	□$_6$喘促明显，但不影响活动	□$_9$喘息不得平卧
胸闷	□$_0$无	□$_3$轻微	□$_6$胸闷明显，但不影响活动	□$_9$胸闷不能活动
心悸	□$_0$无	□$_3$轻微	□$_6$心悸，时作时止	□$_9$持续心悸
口干	□$_0$无	□$_3$轻微	□$_6$口干，偶欲饮水	□$_9$口干，时欲饮水
口苦	□$_0$无	□$_3$偶有口苦	□$_6$常有口苦	□$_9$持续口苦
口渴	□$_0$无	□$_3$口干唇燥	□$_6$口渴	□$_9$口渴喜饮
纳差	□$_0$无	□$_3$轻微	□$_6$尚可进食	□$_9$完全不欲饮食
恶心呕吐	□$_0$无	□$_3$恶心欲吐	□$_6$呕吐	□$_9$频繁呕吐，食入即吐
腹泻	□$_0$无	□$_3$<3次/d	□$_6$4~6次/d	□$_9$>6次/d
便秘	□$_0$无	□$_3$<3 d/次	□$_6$4~6 d/次	□$_9$>6 d/次
失眠	□$_0$无	□$_3$入睡困难	□$_6$入睡困难，易惊醒	□$_9$入睡困难，易惊醒，经常做噩梦
舌象				

附录 3

舌苔拍摄要点

一、嘱患者自然伸舌。患者正面站立或端坐，舌头尽量自然下伸，舌面平展，低于拍摄角度。

二、光线充足柔和。尽量在自然光或者日光灯下面向光线角度拍摄。

三、避免染苔。拍摄时注意避免患者因食物或药物染色对苔色影响。

四、舌体全覆盖。照片拍摄范围通常覆盖鼻孔下方到下颌，需全面展示舌尖、舌面及舌根整体部位。

五、请参照下图拍摄。

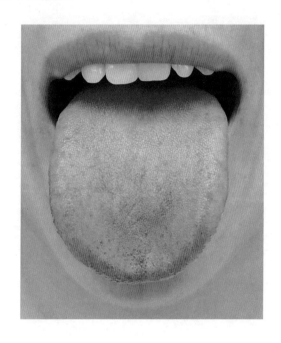

附录 4

参考穴位图

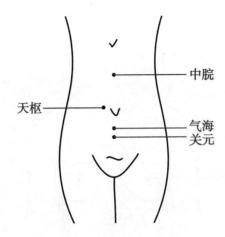

关元：在下腹部，前正中线上，脐中下 3 寸

气海：在下腹部，前正中线上，脐中下 1.5 寸

天枢：在腹中部，距脐中 2 寸

中脘：在上腹部，前正中线上，脐中上 4 寸

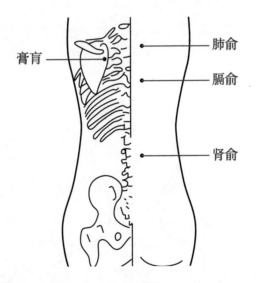

肺俞：在背部，第 3 胸椎棘突下，旁开 1.5 寸

膈俞：在背部，第 7 胸椎棘突下，旁开 1.5 寸

肾俞：在腰部，第 2 腰椎棘突下，旁开 1.5 寸

膏肓：在背部，第 4 胸椎棘突下，旁开 3 寸

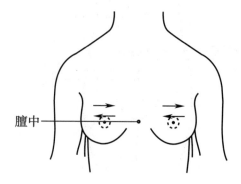

膻中：在胸部，前正中线上，平第 4 肋间，两乳头连线的中点

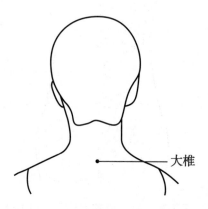

大椎：在后正中线上，第 7 颈椎棘突下凹陷中

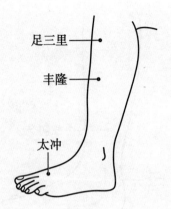

足三里：在小腿前外侧，当犊鼻下 3 寸，距胫骨前缘一横指（中指）

太冲：在足背侧，第 1、2 跖骨间隙的后方凹陷中

丰隆：在小腿前外侧，外踝尖上 8 寸，距胫骨前缘两横指（中指）

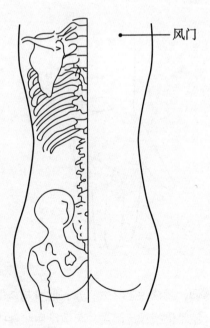

风门：在背部，第 2 胸椎棘突下，旁开 1.5 寸

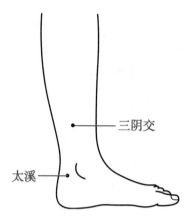

太溪：在足部内踝后方，内踝尖与跟腱之间的凹陷处

三阴交：在小腿内侧，足内踝尖上 3 寸，胫骨内侧缘后方

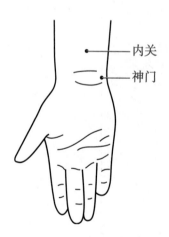

内关：在前臂掌侧，腕横纹上 2 寸，掌长肌腱与桡侧腕屈肌腱之间

神门：在腕部，腕掌侧横纹尺侧端，尺侧腕屈肌腱桡侧凹陷处

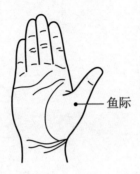

鱼际

鱼际：在手拇指末节（第1掌指关节）后凹陷处，约在第1掌骨中点桡侧赤白肉际处

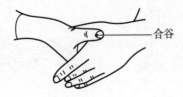

合谷

合谷：在手背，第1、2掌骨间，当第二掌骨桡侧的中点处。

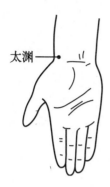

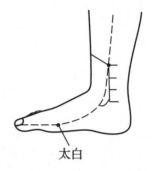

太渊：人体腕掌侧横纹桡侧，桡动脉搏动处。

太白：在足内侧缘，当足大趾本节（第 1 跖趾关节）后下方赤白肉际凹陷处。

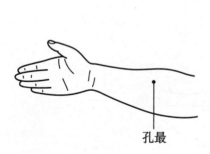

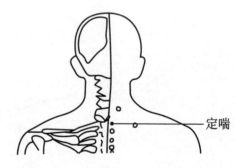

孔最：在前臂掌面桡侧，当尺泽与太渊连线上，腕横纹上 7 寸。

定喘：在背部，当第 7 颈椎棘突下，旁开 0.5 寸。

耳 穴 图

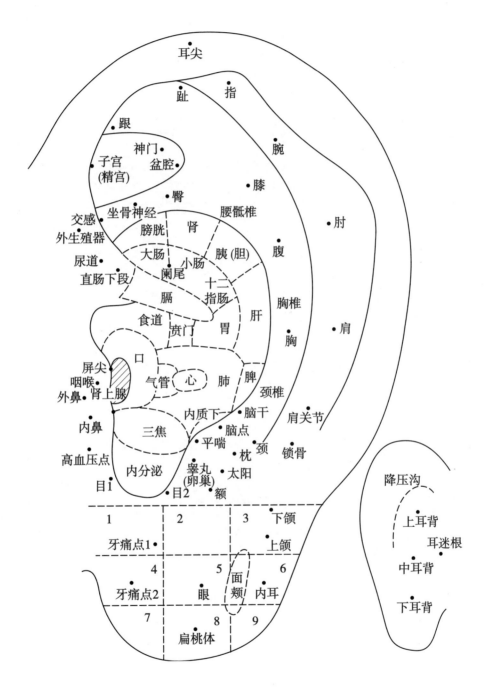

耳屏和对耳屏的内侧面

Compilation Instructions

The COVID-19 pandemic is a major threat to the lives and health of people around the world, as well as a serious challenge to global health security. Since the outbreak, the Chinese government has taken effective measures to control the spread of the epidemic under the direct command of President Xi Jinping. At present, China's situation in epidemic prevention and control remains severe. Tedros Adhanom Ghebreyesus, Director-General of the World Health Organization, pointed out that China's strong measures are not only protecting the Chinese people, but also protecting the people throughout the world. They have bought time for global epidemic prevention and control.

Under the strong leadership of President Xi Jinping and the auspices of Chinese government's health departments, the integrated approach combining traditional Chinese medicine and western medicine has achieved positive and effective results. Traditional Chinese medicine (abbreviated to TCM) is an important part of the integration of Chinese and western medicine. As a national treasure with a very long history, TCM has helped Chinese people defeat countless plagues during the thousands of years of development of the Chinese nation. It has shown good curative effects in the fight against the SARS epidemic in 2003 and against COVID-19 epidemic in China in the past two months. With the support of modern technologies, TCM has played a unique role in the close cooperation with western medicine and proved effective for patients with various symptoms at different stages. According to a press conference by the State Council Information Office on March 23 and Yu Yanhong, the person in charge of the National Administration of Traditional Chinese Medicine, 74,187 of the confirmed cases in China have been treated with traditional Chinese medicine, accounting for 91.5% of the total, and 61,449 patients in Hubei were treated with traditional Chinese medicine, accounting for 90.6%. Clinical observations show that the total effective rate of traditional Chinese medicine reaches more than 90%. None of the mild cases in the group with TCM intervention showed any sign of deterioration; the mortality risk of severe/critical cases in the group to which TCM herbal soups are administered was lowered by more than 80%. Compared with the rate of cured cases relapsing into positive test results of 2.77% in the group with TCM intervention, which in the group without TCM intervention was 15.79%. In terms of safety, efficacy, applicability and economy, the conditions are ripe now for China to promote the protocol of integrated TCM and western medicine around the globe.

The Chinese government and the National Administration of Traditional Chinese Medicine proposed to promote international cooperation in epidemic prevention, facilitate the development of the community of common destiny for all mankind and enhance the international medical community's understanding of China's practices in integration of traditional Chinese medicine and western medicine. In active response to such proposal, and to fulfill its mission (exchanges and mutual learning, sharing with humanity, and building a healthcare community of common destiny), the Sub-society of International Exchanges and Cooperation of China Society of Ethnic Medicines (SECEM) has initiated a special project based on China's experience. The research team of the project is made up of renowned experts in TCM treatment of febrile diseases, management of hospitals for infectious diseases, pharmacology, pharmaceutical preparation, translation and international exchanges from China Academy of Chinese Medical Sciences, Tsinghua University Affiliated Beijing Tsinghua Changgung Hospital, Jiangxi University of Traditional Chinese Medicine, Beijing University of Chinese Medicine, the 8th Medical Center of Chinese PLA General Hospital and other institutions. The team has compiled the *"Diagnosis and Treatment Protocol for COVID-19: An Integrated Approach Combining Chinese and Western Medicine*

Recommended for International Community" based on the clinical experience of front-line experts from Wuhan National TCM Medical Team for COVID-19 and representative provinces by referring to the *"Diagnosis and Treatment Protocol for COVID-19"* issued by the National Health Commission of the PRC and National Administration of Traditional Chinese Medicine, the protocols issued by provincial governments in China, as well as considerations of current global clinical symptoms and relevant international laws. Meanwhile, inputs have been solicited simultaneously from medical experts of Japan, Sweden, Italy, Cuba, Tanzania and Mexico, so as to make the protocol as readable and practical as possible for international peers.

As the therapeutic principle of TCM is "Three Categories of Etiological Factors" (time, location and individuals), this protocol will be continuously updated and optimized to factor in the progress of international cooperation and address the specific cases and needs of the target countries.

Based on our original aspiration of mutual assistance to overcome difficulties and our expectation of mutual reliance and cooperation, we would like to join hands with our counterparts in the international community to make concerted efforts for the ultimate triumph over this biblical contagious disease against the human kind.

1. Background and Basic Idea for Developing the Protocol

The basic idea for developing this protocol is to provide a new approach to the global medical community by bringing together traditional Chinese medicine (TCM) and western medicine, which complement each other's strengths. The protocol fully embodies the in-depth integration of TCM and western medicine based on the review of historical documents about the prevention and treatment of epidemics in China over the past thousands of years, as well as the findings of modern medical research. In addition, the protocol is worked out by referring to the *"Diagnosis and Treatment Protocol for COVID-19"* issued by the National Health Commission of the People's Republic of China and the National Administration of Traditional Chinese Medicine as well as those protocols issued by provincial governments in China, therefore, the protocol is theoretically sound and clinically practical.

2. Main Features of the Protocol

2.1 Universal Language and Unified Expressions

TCM terminologies in the protocol are replaced with modern medical expressions, and the whole protocol has been translated from Chinese into an internationally acceptable language. Accessible to medical professionals of modern medicine, this TCM-based protocol can give full play to the combined effect of traditional Chinese medicine and western medicine.

2.2 A Clear, Modular and Stage-based Layout

To facilitate understanding and operation in different countries, the protocol proposes six stages in the progression of the epidemic situation, namely, prevention, suspected cases, mild and ordinary cases, severe cases, critical cases, and recovery. One basic prescription is recommended for each stage. Depending on the specific symptoms, medications in the protocol are based on syndrome differentiation and combination of Chinese patent medicines. With a modular and sheet-based structure, the protocol is convenient, effective, easy to comprehend and practical.

2.3 Consideration of Three Categories of Etiological Factors (Time, Location and Individuals) for Targeted Treatment

To facilitate accurate diagnosis and medications based on the three factors, the protocol has designed a remote tongue diagnosis and questionnaire for interrogation enquiry to identify the specific symptoms of patients. In this way, the diagnosis is more accurate, the treatment more targeted and effective.

2.4 Following Historical Classics and Scientific Standards

First, the medicines used in the protocol are mainly from classic prescriptions of TCM, which have a long history of application and proven effects, and have accumulated a large amount of Real World Evidence (RWE). In addition, they are based on *Pharmacopoeia of People's Republic of China (Editon 2020)* and ministerial standards in China. Second, the dosage forms are easy to use. Tablets, capsules, granules, oral liquids are the preferred forms, followed by traditional pills, powder and decoctions. These easy-to-use dosage forms make the medicines more acceptable while guaranteeing their clinical effect. Third, the use of raw medicinal materials complies with regulations. To be compliant with the laws and regulations of various countries, the decoctions in the protocol are designed to avoid banned herbs and any materials with potential safety hazards (such as Ephedra and Asarum), as well as any materials derived from endangered or wild animals and plants.

2.5 Collective Wisdom of Chinese and Foreign Experts

The protocol compilation team reflects the integration of TCM and western medicine, the combination of medicine and pharmacy, the integration of multiple disciplines, and the collective wisdom of senior, middle-aged, and young professionals. The team is composed of experts with extensive clinical experience, venerable academicians and nationally renowned veteran doctors of TCM. Moreover, the protocol contains inputs from representatives of medical and pharmaceutical experts from five continents, who fully exchanged their views and carried out discussions.

3. Arrangement of Protocol Compilation and International Dissemination

3.1 Protocol Compilation Instructors

Huang Luqi	President of China Academy of Chinese Medical Sciences, and Academician of Chinese Academy of Engineering
Dong Jiahong	Dean of School of Clinical Medicine, Tsinghua University, President of Tsinghua University Affiliated Beijing Tsinghua Changgung Hospital, and Academician of Chinese Academy of Engineering

3.2 International Promoters

Huang Guifang	Vice-president of Sub-society of International Exchanges and Cooperation of China Society of Ethnic Medicines (SECEM), former Deputy Director of Foreign Affairs Office of the State Council of China, former Director of Secretariat of General Office of the State Council, and former Chinese Ambassador to the Philippines, New Zealand and Zimbabwe
Xu Yicong	Former Chinese Ambassador to Cuba, Argentina and Ecuador, and former Deputy Director-General of Latin America Department of the Ministry of Foreign Affairs

of China

Guo Chongli   Vice-president of Sub-society of International Exchanges and Cooperation of China Society of Ethnic Medicines (SECEM), former Deputy Director-General of the Information Department of the Ministry of Foreign Affairs of China, former Chinese Ambassador to Jamaica and Kenya, and former Representative of China in UNEP and UN Habitat

Zhao Rongxian   Vice-president of Sub-society of International Exchanges and Cooperation of China Society of Ethnic Medicines (SECEM), former Deputy Director-General of Latin America Department of the Ministry of Foreign Affairs of China, and former Chinese Ambassador to Cuba and Venezuela

Wu Sike   Member of the Foreign Policy Advisory Committee of the Ministry of Foreign Affairs of China, Advisory Committee Member of Sub-society of International Exchanges and Cooperation of China Society of Ethnic Medicines (SECEM), former Director-General of the Department of West Asia and North Africa of the Ministry of Foreign Affairs of China, former Chinese Ambassador to Egypt and Saudi Arabia, and China's Special Envoy to the Middle East

Zhou Xiaopei   Advisory Committee Member of Sub-society of International Exchanges and Cooperation of China Society of Ethnic Medicines (SECEM), former Director of the Eurasian Department of the Ministry of Foreign Affairs of China, and former Chinese Ambassador to Ukraine, Poland and Kazakhstan

Fu Yuancong   Advisory Committee Member of Sub-society of International Exchanges and Cooperation of China Society of Ethnic Medicines (SECEM), and former Ambassador Extraordinary and Plenipotentiary of China to East Timor

3.3 TCM Reviewer

Liu Jingyuan   Professor and Doctoral Supervisor of Beijing University of Chinese Medicine, TCM expert in febrile diseases, famous veteran TCM doctor in China

3.4 Finalizer of English Version

Chen Mingming   Chairman of Sub-society of International Exchanges and Cooperation of China Society of Ethnic Medicines (SECEM), member of Advisory Committee on Public Diplomacy of the Ministry of Foreign Affairs of China, former Director of Translation Office of the Ministry of Foreign Affairs of China, and former Chinese Ambassador to New Zealand and to Sweden

3.5 Chief Director

Yang Kai   Executive Vice-president and Secretary General of Sub-society of International Exchanges and Cooperation of China Society of Ethnic Medicines (SECEM)

3.6 Chief Editors

Professor Yang Ming	Doctoral Supervisor and Vice-president of Jiangxi University of Traditional Chinese Medicine, and pharmaceutical scientist of TCM
Professor Bu Haibing	Vice-president of former 309 Hospital, Senior Engineer, and expert of hospital management and health technology
Professor Zhu Xiaoxin	Doctoral Supervisor, former Party Secretary and Associate Director of Institute of Chinese Materia Medica, China Academy of Chinese Medical Sciences, and pharmacologist of TCM

3.7 Associate Editors-in-Chief

Professor Li Hao	Leader of National TCM Medical Team of Wuhan Jinyintan Hospital, and Vice-president of Xiyuan Hospital of China Academy of Chinese Medical Sciences
Professor Lin Minggui	Expert of Central Health Care Committee, and Leader of COVID-19 Expert Team and Director of Infection Department of Tsinghua University Affiliated Beijing Tsinghua Changgung Hospital
Professor Liu Liangji	Doctoral Supervisor, Vice-president of Affiliated Hospital of China Jiangxi University of Traditional Chinese

Medicine, and Expert Team Leader
for Jiangxi Province COVID-19 TCM
Prevention and Treatment

3.8 Editorial Board Members

Zhou Bugao	Professor, Jiangxi University of Traditional Chinese Medicine
Zhang Yuanbing	Professor and Chief TCM Physician, Jiangxi University of Traditional Chinese Medicine
Lan Zhihui	Professor and Chief TCM Physician, Jiangxi University of Traditional Chinese Medicine
Song Minxian	Professor, Jiangxi University of Traditional Chinese Medicine
Li Shouzhang	Associate Chief TCM Physician of China Sweden TCM Treatment Center, China Qingdao Hospital of Integrated Traditional Chinese and Western Medicine, and Huarui Herun TCM Institution
Qin Chengwei	Leader of China-dispatched Tanzania Medical Team, and Chief Physician of Affiliated Hospital of China Binzhou Medical College
Jia Qingliang	President of Nepal Chinese Hospital
Zhu Ming	President of Zhongfang Red Cross International Hospital, Hunan Province, China
Zhang Rong	Associate Professor of Peking University
Zhang Leichang	Associate Professor and Associate Chief TCM Physician, Jiangxi University of Traditional Chinese Medicine
Ding Zhaohui	Lecturer and Attending TCM Physician, Jiangxi

	University of Traditional Chinese Medicine
Li Mingdi	AHPRA Registered TCM Practitioner, and Doctoral Student (majoring in Complementary Medicine) of Royal Melbourne Institute of Technology University

3.9 English Translators

Li Taoan	College of Humanities, Jiangxi University of Traditional Chinese Medicine, China
Yu Yawei	College of Humanities, Jiangxi University of Traditional Chinese Medicine, China
Ren Junwei	College of Humanities, Jiangxi University of Traditional Chinese Medicine, China
Tu Yuming	College of Humanities, Jiangxi University of Traditional Chinese Medicine, China
Zheng Hongxiang	College of Humanities, Jiangxi University of Traditional Chinese Medicine, China
Yang Jurong	College of Humanities, Jiangxi University of Traditional Chinese Medicine, China
Chen Zhiyuan	College of Humanities, Jiangxi University of Traditional Chinese Medicine, China

Diagnosis and Treatment Protocol for COVID-19: An Integrated Approach Combining Chinese and Western Medicine Recommended for International Community

1. Clinical Manifestations and Characteristics

According to the current epidemiological investigations, the incubation period of COVID-19 ranges from 1 to 14 days and mostly from 3 to 7 days.

Fever, dry cough and fatigue are considered the main clinical manifestations. Some patients present with symptoms such as aversion to cold, stuffy and runny nose, headache, pharyngalgia, myalgia, muscular pain, joint pain, reduced appetite, dry and sticky mouth, anidrosis, diarrhea, dry stool, etc. In severe cases, dyspnea and/or hypoxemia usually occurs one week after the onset of disease, and some patients can rapidly progress to acute respiratory distress syndrome, septic shock, intractable metabolic acidosis, hemorrhage and coagulation dysfunction. It is worth noting that severely or critically-ill patients may have a moderate or low fever or no fever at all.

Some patients may only have light fever, mild fatigue and so on, and show no sign of pneumonia. Most of them usually recover after one week, but are still contagious.

Most of the patients have a favorable prognosis, but some of them turn severely or critically ill. The elderly and people with chronic underlying diseases usually have poor prognosis while symptoms of children are relatively mild.

2. Laboratory Examination

2.1 General Examination

In the early stage of COVID-19, a normal or decreased total white blood cell count and a decreased lymphocyte count can be found in patients. In addition, increased value of transaminase, LDH, muscle enzymes and myoglobin can occur in some patients; and raised level of troponin can be seen in some critically ill patients. In most cases, the laboratory test shows a raised C-reactive protein value and erythrocyte sedimentation rate but a normal procalcitonin value. Among severe patients, D-dimer value increased and peripheral blood lymphocytes decreased persistently. In addition, elevated values of inflammatory factors can often be seen in severe and critical patients.

2.2 Etiological and Serological Examination

2.2.1 Etiological examination: The nucleic acid of COVID-19 can be detected in nasopharyngeal swabs, sputum, and other specimens like lower respiratory tract secretion, blood and feces by RT-PCR and/or NGS. Detection of lower respiratory tract specimens (sputum or airway extracts) can provide more accurate evidence for diagnosis. All the specimens collected should be sent and tested as soon as possible.

2.2.2 Serological examination: The COVID-19 specific IgM antibodies mostly become positive 3 to 5 days after the onset, and the patients may show a ⩾4-fold rise in IgG antibody titer between the acute and convalescent stages.

2.3 Chest Radiography

In the early stage of COVID-19, the images show that there are multiple small patched shadows and interstitial changes, especially in the lung periphery. As the disease progresses, the images of these patients further develop into multiple ground glass shadows and infiltration shadows in both lungs. In severe cases, lung consolidation may occur. Pleural effusion is rarely seen in patients with COVID-19.

3. Diagnostic Standards

3.1 Suspected Cases

Comprehensive analysis is conducted based on the epidemic history and clinical manifestations described below.

3.1.1 Epidemiological History

(1) Experience of traveling or living in an epidemic-stricken area or its surrounding areas, or a community where a case has been reported within 14 days before the onset.

(2) Contact with patients infected by COVID-19 within 14 days before the onset.

(3) Contact with patients of fever or respiratory symptoms from epidemic-stricken area or a community where a case has been reported within 14 days before the onset.

(4) Clustering cases (two or more cases with fever and/or respiratory symptoms emerge within 2 weeks within a small group, like family, office, and classroom).

3.1.2 Clinical Manifestations

(1) Fever and/or respiratory symptoms.

(2) Radiographic features of COVID-19.

(3) In the early stage, the total number of white blood cell and the count of lymphocyte can be normal or decreased.

The suspected case can be identified when an individual has any one of the epidemiological histories plus any two of the clinical manifestations mentioned above, or an individual has no clear epidemiological history but have all the three clinical manifestations.

3.2 Confirmed Cases

Suspected cases that show any one of the following etiological or serological evidences can be confirmed.

3.2.1 The COVID-2019 nucleic acid test through real-time fluorescence RT-PCR produces a positive result.

3.2.2 The virus gene sequence is highly homologous to the known COVID-2019.

3.2.3 The COVID-2019 specific IgM antibody and IgG antibody in the serum are positive. The novel coronavirus specific IgG antibody in the serum turns positive, or the patients show a ≥4-fold rise in IgG antibody titer between the acute and convalescent stages.

4. Differential Diagnosis

4.1 The mild COVID-2019 infected cases should be differentiated from those of upper respiratory tract infections caused by other viruses.

4.2 It should be mainly differentiated from viral pneumonia caused by influenza virus, adenovirus or respiratory syncytial virus, and mycoplasma pneumonia. Methods including rapid antigen detection and multiple PCR nucleic acid test should be adopted to test common respiratory pathogens, especially for suspected cases.

4.3 It should be also distinguished from non-infectious diseases like vasculitis, dermatomyositis, and organizing pneumonia.

5. Recommended Preventive Interventions

Indications: People with insufficient immunity and the elderly with weak constitution among general population.

Cautions: It is forbidden for pregnant women. If there is any discomfort after the medicine is taken, stop the medication in time (Table 1).

Table 1　Preventive Prescriptions

Master Prescription	Concomitant Symptom	Additive Prescription
Kuangfu Zhengqi San (Healthy-Qi-Supporting Tea) (Annex 1-1) Dosage form: teabag (20 mesh), 5g / bag. Administration: 1 bag at a time, twice a day, for a week, taken orally after mixed with boiled water, or decocted in 250ml water for 5 minutes. Or Yupingfeng (Jade Screen) Oral Liquid (Annex 1-2).	Gastrointestinal discomfort	Huoxiang Zhengqi Shui (Agastache Qi-Rectifying Oral Liquid) (Annex 1-3), Huoxiang Zhengqi Wan (Agastache Qi-Rectifying Pill) (Annex 1-4, 1-5, 1-6)
	Fever with lack of strength	Xiaochaihu (Minor Bupleurum) Granule (Annex 1-7), Qingre Bawei (Heat-Clearing Eight-Ingredients) Capsule (Annex 1-8), Lianhua Qingwen (Forsythia Honeysuckle Epidemic-Cleaning) Capsule/Granule (Annex 1-9, 1-10), or Jinhua Qinggan (Honeysuckle Cold-Clearing) Granule (Annex 1-11)
	Systemic soreness and pain	Jiuwei Qianghuo Wan (Nine-Ingredients Notopterygium Pill) (Annex 1-12) or Chuanxiong Chatiao (Ligusticum Tea-Making) Granule (Annex 1-13)
	Cough	Tongxuan Lifei Wan (Lung-Ventilating-Dredging-Rectifying Pill) (Annex 1-14, 1-15)
	Chest oppression	Guilong Kechuanning Pian (Cinnamon-Twig Dragon-Bone Cough-Panting-Calming Tablet) (Annex 1-16)
	Cough with yellow phlegm	Xianzhuli (Fresh Bamboo Juice) Oral Liquid(Annex 1-17)
	Sore throat or dry throat	Yinqiao Jiedu Wan (Honeysuckle Forsythia Toxin-Resolving Pill) (Annex 1-18)
	Constipation	Sanhuang Pian (Scutellaria Coptis Phellodendron Tablet) (Annex 1-19)
	Dry throat or tongue, or thirst	Baihe Gujin Wan (Lily Metal-Securing Pill) (Annex 1-20, 1-21)
	Insomnia	Anshen Buxin Liuwei Wan (Spirit-Calming Heart-Tonifying Six-Ingredients Pill) (Annex 1-22)

Recommended therapies of acupuncture and moxibustion, acupuncture with electric stimulation as well as transcutaneous acupoint electrical stimulation.

Their conventional practices can help improve immunity.

Selected Acupoints: Zusanli (ST36) (both sides), Qihai (CV6), Zhongwan (CV12). If filiform needle is adopted, retain the needle for 25-30 minutes each time for the acupuncture reinforcing purpose. If electric needle or transcutaneous acupoint electrical stimulation is adopted, select the low frequency of 2 Hz and an electric current strength of 10-20 mA and retain the needle for 15-20 minutes each time, once every other day.

6. Syndrome Differentiation and Treatment

6.1 Prevention and Treatment of Suspected Cases (Table 2)

Table 2   Preventive and Treatment Prescriptions for Suspected Cases

Master Prescription	Concomitant Symptom	Additive Prescription
Yupingfeng (Jade Screen) Oral Liquid (Annex 1-2)	Gastrointestinal discomfort, pale tongue with teeth marks or light red tongue, white Thick putrid slimy tongue coating or white slimy coating	Huoxiang Zhengqi Shui (Agastache Qi-Rectifying Oral Liquid) (Annex 1-3) Huoxiang Zhengqi Wan (Agastache Qi-Rectifying Pill) (Annex 1-4, 1-5, 1-6)
	Fever, lack of strength, pale tongue or light red tongue, white slimy coating	Xiaochaihu (Minor Bupleurum) Granule (Annex 1-7), or Qingre Bawei (Heat-Clearing Eight-Ingredients) Capsule (Annex 1-8)
	Systemic soreness and pain, pale tongue or light red tongue, white slimy coating	Jiuwei Qianghuo Wan (Nine-Ingredients Notopterygium Pill) (Annex 1-12) or Chuanxiong Chatiao (Ligusticum Tea-Making) Granule (Annex 1-13)

Master Prescription	Concomitant Symptom	Additive Prescription
Yupingfeng (Jade Screen) Oral Liquid (Annex 1-2)	Cough, pale tongue or light red tongue, white thick slimy tongue coating or white slimy coating	Tongxuan Lifei Wan (Lung-Ventilating-Dredging-Rectifying Pill) (Annex 1-14, 1-15)
	Chest oppression, pale tongue or light red tongue, white thick slimy tongue coating or white slimy coating	Guilong Kechuanning Pian (Cinnamon-Twig Dragon-Bone Cough-Panting-Calming Tablet) (Annex 1-16)
	Cough with yellow phlegm, red tongue, yellow slimy tongue coating	Xianzhuli (Fresh Bamboo Juice) Oral Liquid (Annex 1-17)
	Sore throat or dry throat, red tongue, thin yellow tongue coating	Yinqiao Jiedu Wan (Honeysuckle Forsythia Toxin-Resolving Pill) (Annex 1-18)
	Constipation, red tongue, yellow thick tongue coating	Sanhuang Pian (Scutellaria Coptis Phellodendron Tablet) (Annex 1-19)
	Dry throat, thirsty, dry tongue with scanty fluids	Baihe Gujin Wan (Lily Metal-Securing Pill) (Annex 1-20, 1-21)
	Insomnia, red tongue, thin white tongue coating	Anshen Buxin Liuwei Wan (Spirit-Calming Heart-Tonifying Six-Ingredients Pill) (Annex 1-22)

6.2 Mild and Common Syndromes (for suspected cases, please refer to the treatment plans for mild and common syndromes)

6.2.1 TCM Syndrome Differentiation and Treatment

(1) Cold Dampness Syndrome (Table 3)

Clinical manifestations: Low fever (37.3 ℃≤ T ≤ 38.0 ℃), fatigue, systemic soreness and pain, coughing, expectoration, chest oppression, suffocation, poor appetite, nausea, vomiting, sticky unsmooth stool, pale tongue with teeth marks or light red tongue, white thick putrid slimy tongue coating or white slimy coating, soggy or slippery pulse.

Table 3   Prescriptions for Mild and Common Cold Dampness Syndromes

Master Prescription	Concomitant Symptom	Additive Prescription
Huoxiang Zhengqi Wan/Shui (Agastache Qi-Rectifying Pill/ Oral Liquid) (Annex 1-3, 1-4, 1-5, 1-6)	Fever	Xiaochaihu (Minor Bupleurum) Granule(Annex 1-7)
	Systemic soreness and pain	Jiuwei Qianghuo Wan (Nine-Ingredients Notopterygium Pill) (Annex 1-12) or Chuanxiong Chatiao (Ligusticum Tea-Making) Granule (Annex 1-13)
	Cough	Tongxuan Lifei Wan (Lung-Ventilating-Dredging-Rectifying Pill) (Annex 1-14, 1-15)
	Chest oppression	Guilong Kechuanning Pian (Cinnamon-Twig Dragon-Bone Cough-Panting-Calming Tablet) (Annex 1-16)

(2) Damp Heat Syndrome (Table 4)

Clinical manifestations: Low fever (37.3 ℃ ≤ T≤ 38.0 ℃) or no fever, slight aversion to cold, fatigue, head and body heaviness, muscle soreness and pain, dry cough with scanty phlegm, sore throat, dry mouth without desire to drink, or accompanied with chest oppression and gastric stuffiness, no sweat or unsmooth sweating, or nausea, vomiting, poor appetite, mild diarrhea or sticky unsmooth stool, light red tongue, white thick slimy tongue coating or thin yellow coating, slippery rapid pulse or soggy pulse.

Table 4   Prescriptions for Mild and Common Damp Heat Syndromes

Master Prescription	Concomitant Symptom	Additive Prescription
Qingre Bawei (Heat-Clearing Eight-Ingredients) Capsule (Annex 1-8)	Cough with yellow phlegm	Xianzhuli (Fresh Bamboo Juice) Oral Liquid (Annex 1-17)
	Sore throat or dry throat	Yingqiao Jiedu Wan (Honeysuckle Forsythia Toxin-Resolving Pill) (Annex 1-18)
	Constipation	Sanhuang Pian (Scutellaria Coptis Phellodendron Tablet) (Annex 1-19)
	Insomnia and anxiety	Anshen Buxin Liuwei Wan (Spirit-Calming Heart-Tonifying Six-Ingredients Pill) (Annex 1-22)

(3) For the above suspected cases, and cases with mild and common syndrome, the recommended treatment formula is as follows:

1) Jiedu Yiqi San (Toxin-Resolving Qi-Enriching Tea) (Annex 1-23)

Dosage form: Teabag (20 mesh), 5g / bag;

Administration: 3 bags at a time, 3 times a day, for three days, taken orally after it is mixed with boiled water, or decocted in 250ml water for 5 minutes.

2) Qingfei Paidu Tang (Lung-Clearing Toxin-Expelling Decoction)

3) Huashi Baidu (Dampness-Resolving Toxin Defeating) Granule (Annex 1-24)

4) Therapies of acupuncture and moxibustion, acupuncture with electric stimulation as well as transcutaneous acupoint electrical stimulation.

Selected Acupoints: Hegu (LI4) (both sides), Zusanli (ST36) (both sides), Taichong (LR3) (both sides), Shenque (CV8). If filiform needle is adopted, retain the needle for 25-30 minutes each time for reinforcing-reducing purposes. If electric needle or transcutaneous acupoint electrical stimulation is adopted, select the low frequency of 2 Hz and an electric current strength of 10-20 mA and retain the needle for 15-20 minutes each time, once every day.

6.2.2 Basic Treatment

(1) Advise the patient to rest in bed, strengthen supportive treatment, and ensure adequate nutrition; pay attention to water and electrolyte balance to maintain internal environment stability; closely monitor vital signs, oxygen saturation (of finger tip), etc.

(2) As required by the patient's conditions, monitor blood and urine routine, CRP, and biochemical indicators (transaminase, myocardial enzyme, kidney function, etc.), coagulation function, arterial blood gas analysis, chest radiography, etc.

(3) Patients with symptoms of chest tightness and wheezing or hypoxemia should be provided with timely and effective oxygen treatment, including oxygen inhalation through nasal catheter or facemask, and high-flow nasal catheter oxygen therapy.

6.2.3 Antiviral Treatment

To date, there is still no proven treatment for COVID-19. Try to administer alpha-interferon (with 2ml of sterile water for injection added each time, in aerosol form taken by inhalation, twice per day, at a dose of 5 million units or equivalent dosage each time for adults), ribavirin (500 mg for adults each time, 2-3 injections per day intravenously; the course of treatment should be no more than 10 days), chloroquine phosphate (for adults aged from 18 to 65: if the body weight is more than 50kg, the treatment lasts for 7 days, twice a day, 500mg each time; if the body weight is less than 50kg, the treatment can be given twice a day, 500mg each time on the first 2 days, and 500mg only once a day from the third to the seventh day).

Be aware of adverse reactions and contraindications of these drugs (e.g., chloroquine is forbidden for heart patients) and such problems as side-effects caused by the combined use of them with other drugs. The efficacy of the drugs used above should be further assessed in clinical application. It is not recommended to use 3 or more antiviral drugs at one time, and related drugs should be stopped and symptomatic treatment should be given immediately if intolerable toxic and side effects occur.

6.2.4 Antibiotic Therapy

Avoid abuse or inappropriate use of antibiotic agents, especially combined application of broad-spectrum antibiotic agents. When WBC is >10,000 and/or N (neutrophil) is >85%, antibiotic therapy can be considered, and the course of the therapy is generally 5-7 days. Antibiotics should be selected according to the specific clinical situations.

6.3 Severe Cases

6.3.1 Clinical Warning Indicators of Severe and Critical Cases

(1) Adults

① Progressive decline of peripheral blood lymphocytes.

② Progressive increase of peripheral blood inflammatory factors such as Il-6, and c-reactive protein.

③ Progressive increase of lactic acid.

④ Rapid progress of lung lesions in a short period.

(2) Children

① Increase of respiratory rate.

② Poor mental reaction and lethargy.

③ Progressive increase of lactic acid.

④ Chest radiography shows bilateral or multi-lobe infiltration, pleural effusion or rapid progression of lesions in a short period.

⑤ Infants under the age of months or those suffering from underlying diseases (congenital heart disease, bronchopulmonary dysplasia, respiratory tract malformation, abnormal hemoglobin, severe malnutrition, etc.), or immune deficiency or hypoimmunity (long-term use of immunosuppressive agents).

6.3.2 TCM Syndrome Differentiation and Treatment

(1) Syndrome of Epidemic Toxin Blocking the Lung

Clinical manifestations: fever with red face (38.0 ℃<T≤ 39.0 ℃), cough, yellow sticky, and less phlegm, or phlegm with blood, wheezing and shortness of breath (RR>30 breaths/min); or oxygen saturation of finger tip≤93% in a resting state; or arterial partial pressure of oxygen (PaO$_2$)/Fraction of inspiration of oxygen (FiO$_2$) ≤300mmHg; or chest radiography shows rapid progression of lung lesions within 24-48 hours (>50%); fatigue, dry, bitter and sticky mouth, nausea and loss of appetite, inhibited defecation, scanty dark urine, red tongue, yellow slimy tongue coating, and slippery rapid pulse.

Recommended Chinese patent medicine: Niuhuang Qingxin Wan (Annex 1-25) (Bezoar Heart-Clearing Pill) or Qingre Bawei (Heat-Clearing Eight-Ingredients) Capsule.

(2) Syndrome of Flaring Heat in Qi and Blood Aspects(Table 5)

Clinical manifestations: High fever, dysphoria and thirst (T> 39.0℃), wheezing and shortness of breath (RR>30 breaths/min); or oxygen saturation of finger tip≤93% in a resting state; or arterial partial pressure of oxygen (PaO$_2$)/ Fraction of inspiration of oxygen (FiO$_2$) ≤300mmHg; or chest radiography shows rapid progression of lung lesions within 24-48 hours (>50%), delirium, gibberish, blurred vision, or subcutaneous bleeding or vomiting blood, or limb convulsions, purple tongue with little or no coating, sunken, deep thready and rapid pulse, or floating, large and rapid pulse.

Table 5　Prescriptions for Severe Syndromes of Flaring Heat in Qi and Blood Aspects

Master Prescription	Concomitant Symptom	Additive Prescription
Angong Niuhuang Wan (Heart-Calming Bezoar Pill) (Annex 1-26) and Pianzaihuang (made of Bezoar, musk, etc.) (Annex 1-27)	Cough	Tongxuan Lifei Wan (Lung-Ventilating-Dredging-Rectifying Pill) (Annex 1-14, 1-15)
	Dyspnea and sweating	Shengmaiyin (Pulse-Invigorating) Oral Liquid (Annex 1-28)
	Excessive and yellow phlegm	Xianzhuli (Fresh Bamboo Juice) Oral Liquid (Annex 1-17)
	Hemoptysis	Yunnan Baiyao (mainly made of panax pseudo-ginseng of Yunnan Province) (Annex 1-29)

6.3.3 Basic Treatment

(1) Oxygen Therapy

(2) The old and infirm can be provided with the γ-globulin therapy for 3-5 days.

(3) Nutritional supportive treatment should be selected appropriately according to the biochemical indicators.

6.3.4 Chinese Medicinal Injections

(1) Indications: Low or high fever. 5% GS or 0.9% NS 100-250ml combined with Xiyanping Injection (Annex 1-30) (Happiness Inflammation-Deleting Injection) 50-100ml can be given twice a day through intravenous infusion.

(2) Indications: Yellow phlegm, or fever. 5% GS or 0.9% NS 100-250ml combined with Tanreqing Injection (Annex 1-31) (Phlegm-Heat-Clearing Injection) 20-40ml can be given once a day through intravenous infusion.

(3) Indications: High fever and delirium. 5% GS or 0.9% NS 100-250ml combined with Xingnaojing Injection (Annex 1-32) (Brain-Waking-Calming

Injection) 20-40ml can be given once a day through intravenous infusion.

(4) Indications: Chest radiography shows the characteristics of COVID-19. Combine 0.9% NS 100 and Xuebijing Injection (Annex 1-33) (Blood-Must-Be-Clear Injection) 50ml to give additional treatment twice a day through intravenous infusion. If necessary, the combination of the above injections can be considered.

(5) Indications: The presence of immunosuppression. 0.9% Sodium Chloride Injection 250ml plus Shenmai (Ginseng Ophiopogon) Injection (Annex 1-34) 100ml can be given twice a day.

(6) Indication: Shock. 0.9% Sodium Chloride Injection 250ml plus Shenfu Injection (Annex 1-35) (Ginseng Aconite Injection) 100ml can be given twice a day.

6.3.5 Symptomatic Treatment

(1) Fever: For the temperature ⩾38.5℃, Chaihu (Bupleurum) Injection (Annex 1-36) can be given 1-3 times a day, 4ml each time, or Celecoxib (1-2 times a day, 0.2g each time) or Diclofenac Sodium Suppositories (1-2 times a day, 25mg-50mg each time);

(2) Cough: Dextromethorphan (3-4 times a day, 15-30mg each time), or Robitussin (3-4 times a day, 10ml each time) can be given;

(3) Excessive phlegm and difficulty to cough it up: Ambroxol (3-4 times a day, 30mg each time), or Acetylcysteine Effervescent Tablets (1-3 times a day, 0.6g each time);

(4) Dyspnea with wheezing in the lung: Theophylline Sustained Release Tablets can be given 2 times a day, 1-2 tablets each time;

(5) Diarrhea: Mengtuoshi San (Smectite Tea) (Annex 1-37) can be administered 3 times a day, 1-2 bags each time.

6.3.6 Application of Antibiotics

Indication: With manifestation of bacterial infection, e.g. WBC> 10,000 and/or neutrophil >85%, antibiotics can be considered for the treatment, generally for 5-7 days. Antibiotics can be selected according to the specific clinical situations.

For example: 0.9% NS100ml and Cefoperazone or Tazobactam 3g are infused intravenously, 2-3 times a day, and/or 0.9% NS100ml and Moxifloxacin 0.4g, once a day; or 0.9% NS100ml and Meropenem 1.0g are infused intravenously 3 times a day (once every 8 hours).

6.3.7 Application of Antiviral Drugs

Try to administer alpha-interferon in aerosol form (with 2ml of sterile water for injection added each time, twice per day, at a dose of 5 million units each time for adults), ribavirin (500mg for adults each time, 2-3 injections per day intravenously); chloroquine phosphate (500mg each time for adults, twice per day). The course of treatment should be no more than 10 days.

6.3.8 Application of Hormone

In principle, application of the hormone should be avoided or used with caution. If it cannot be substituted, it should be used for a short-term period (3-5 days). The recommended dosage should be no more than the equivalent of Methylprednisolone, 1-2mg/(kg · d) Indications of application: significant dyspnea, severe hypoxemia, marked progression of lung lesion monitored by chest radiography, and/or obvious rise of inflammatory indicators.

6.3.9 Treatment of Children

Children who meet any of the following criteria can receive syndrome-based treatment according to adult standards.

(1) Shortness of breath (<2 months old, RR⩾60 breaths/min; 2-12 months old, RR⩾50 breaths/min; 1-5 years old, RR⩾40 breaths/min; >5 years old, RR⩾30 breaths/min), excluding the influence of fever and crying.

(2) Oxygen saturation of finger tip ≤92% in a resting state.

(3) Assisted respiration (moaning, flapping of nose wing, three depressions sign), cyanosis, intermittent apnea.

(4) Drowsiness and convulsions.

(5) Food resistance or feeding difficulties, with signs of dehydration.

6.4 Critical Cases

Clinical manifestations: Difficult breathing, easy panting (mechanical ventilation is needed), abnormal state of consciousness (ICU treatment is needed when shock or failure of another organ occurs), agitation, sweating, cold limbs, dark purple tongue, thick slimy or dry coating, and floating large rootless pulse.

6.4.1 Therapeutic principle: Complications should be actively prevented and treated on the basis of symptomatic treatment; underlying diseases should be treated to avoid secondary infection; support for organ function should be provided in a timely manner.

6.4.2 TCM Syndrome Differentiation and Treatment

Syndrome of Internal Block and External Collapse(Table 6)

Clinical manifestations: Difficult breathing, easy panting or a need for mechanical ventilation, coma, agitation, sweating, cold limbs, dark purple tongue, thick slimy or dry coating, and floating large rootless pulse.

Table 6   Prescriptions for Critical Syndromes of Internal Block and External Collapse

Master Prescription	Concomitant Symptom	Additive Prescription
Shengmaiyin (Pulse-Invigorating) Oral Liquid (Annex 1-28)	Coma with reddened complexion, fever, yellow coating on the tongue, and rapid pulse	Angong Niuhuang Wan (Heart-Calming Bezoar Pill, top choice for concomitant high fever) (Annex 1-26)
	Coma with bluish complexion, cool body, white coating on the tongue, and slow pulse	Suhexiang Wan (Liquidambar Pill) (Annex 1-38)

6.4.3 Usage of Chinese medicinal injection, antibiotics and hormones: the same as the application in the severe cases (6.3).

6.4.4 Respiratory Support

(1) Oxygen therapy: Severe patients should be provided with oxygen inhalation through nasal catheter or facemask, and receive timely assessment about whether respiratory distress and/or hypoxemia are relieved.

(2) High-flow nasal catheter oxygen therapy or non-invasive mechanical ventilation: When respiratory distress and/or hypoxemia cannot be relieved after standard oxygen therapy, high-flow nasal catheter oxygen therapy or non-invasive ventilation should be considered. If the condition does not improve or even worsens within a short period of time (1-2 hours), endotracheal intubation and invasive mechanical ventilation should be performed promptly.

(3) Invasive mechanical ventilation: Lung protective ventilation strategies are adopted, which means to maintain small tidal volume (6-8ml/kg ideal body weight) and low airway platform pressure ($\leqslant 30cmH_2O$) for mechanical ventilation to reduce ventilator-related lung injury. When the platform pressure is $\leqslant 35cmH_2O$, high PEEP can be used appropriately to keep the airway warm and humid; avoid prolonged sedation, and wake up patients early to perform pulmonary

resuscitation. Patient-ventilator asynchrony may occur to many patients, and sedative and muscle relaxants should be used in time; closed sputum suction is selected on basis of the airway secretions, and if necessary, bronchoscopy should be performed, and corresponding treatment adopted.

(4) Salvage treatment: Lung recruitment maneuver is recommended for patients with severe ARDS. If possible, prone position ventilation should be performed for more than 12 hours per day. For those with poor outcome from prone position ventilation, extracorporeal membrane pulmonary oxygenation (ECMO) should be considered as soon as possible if conditions permit. Related indications: ① When FiO_2 exceeds 90%, the oxygenation index is less than 80mmHg, which lasts for more than 3-4 hours; ② Airway platform pressure ≥35cmH$_2$O. For patients with simple respiratory failure, the VV-ECMO mode is preferred; if circulatory support is required, the VA-ECMO mode is used. Weaning trials can begin when the underlying disease is under control and cardiopulmonary function shows signs of recovery.

(5) Circulation Support

Doctors should improve the patient's microcirculation on the basis of adequate fluid resuscitation, administrate vasoactive drugs, closely monitor changes in patients' blood pressure, heart rate, and urine output, lactic acid and alkali residuals in arterial blood gas analysis, and carry out noninvasive or invasive haemodynamic monitoring (if necessary), including echo Doppler, echocardiography, invasive blood pressure or continuous cardiac output (PiCCO). In the treatment process, attention should be paid to the liquid balance to avoid overdose or underdose. If the heart rate of patient is suddenly increased or the blood pressure of patient is suddenly decreased by 20% of the base value, accompanied by symptoms such as poor skin perfusion and decreased urine output, we should closely observe whether the patient has septic shock, gastrointestinal bleeding or heart failure.

(6) Treatment for Renal Failure and Renal Replacement

The causes of renal impairment in critical cases should be understood, such as hypoperfusion and drugs. For the treatment of patients with renal failure, attention should be paid to body fluid balance, acid-base balance and electrolyte balance. In addition, due attention should be given to nitrogen balance, calories and trace elements supplement in nutritional support treatment. Continuous renal replacement therapy (CRRT) can be applied in severe patients, whose indications include: ① hyperkalemia; ② acidosis; ③ pulmonary edema or excessive water load; ④ fluid management in the case of multiple organ dysfunction.

(7) Blood Purification Treatment

The blood purification system includes plasma exchange, absorption, perfusion, blood/plasma filtration, etc., which can remove inflammatory factors and block the "Cytokine Storm", thereby reducing the damage of the inflammatory response to the body. It can be used in the early and mid-term treatment of cytokine storm in severe and critical cases.

(8) Immunotherapy

Tocilizumab can be used for patients with extensive lung lesions (both lungs), severe cases, and those with elevated IL-6 levels in laboratory testing. The first dosage should be 4 to 8 mg/kg and the recommended dosage is 400mg, diluted to 100ml with 0.9% saline, and infused longer than 1 hour. If the first administration is not effective, it can be applied once more after 12 hours (with the same dosage as before). Tocilizumab can be administered for no more than 2 doses, each no more than 800mg. Beware of allergic reactions, and do not use this therapy for people with active infection such as tuberculosis.

(9) Other Treatments

Glucocorticoids can be used appropriately for a short period of time (3-5 days) for patients with deterioration of oxygenation index, rapid progress of lung lesions shown by chest radiography and over activation of inflammatory reaction. Recommended dosage should not exceed 1-2mg/(kg · d) methylprednisolone. It should be noted that a higher dosage of glucocorticoids would delay coronavirus clearance due to immunosuppressive effects; Xuebijing Injection (Blood-Must-Be-Clear Injection) can be given intravenously 100ml each time, twice a day; Intestinal Microecological Preparation can be used to maintain intestinal microecological balance.

Intravenous drip of gamma globulin may be considered as an appropriate treatment in severe and critical cases of children. Pregnant women should decidedly terminate their pregnancy, and a cesarean delivery is preferred.

Anxiety and fear usually occur in many patients; therefore psychological counseling should be strengthened.

7. Convalescence

7.1 TCM Syndrome Differentiation and Treatment

7.1.1 Syndrome of Lung and Spleen Qi Deficiency(Table 7)

Clinical manifestations: Shortness of breath, tiredness, debilitation, poor appetite, nausea, vomiting, abdominal fullness and distension, atonic constipation, mild diarrhea or sticky unsmooth stool, pale enlarged tongue, and white slimy tongue coating.

Table 7　Prescriptions for Convalescent Cases with Syndrome of
Lung and Spleen Qi Deficiency

Master Prescription	Concomitant Symptom	Additive Prescription
Shenling Baizhu San (Codnopsis Poria Ovate Atractylodes Tea) (Annex 1-39), or Shenling Baizhu Wan (Codnopsis Poria Ovate Atractylodes Pill) (Annex 1-40), or Buzhong Yiqi Wan (Middle-Supplementing Qi-Enriching Pill) (Annex 1-41), or Xiangsha Liujun Wan (Cyperus Amomum Six-Gentlemen Pill) (Annex 1-42)	Depression, emotional stress	Xiaoyao Wan (Care-Free Pill) (Annex 1-43)

7.1.2 Syndrome of Dual Deficiency of Qi and Yin(Table 8)

Clinical manifestations: Fatigue, shortness of breath, dry and sticky mouth, palpitation, excessive sweating, low or no fever, dry cough with scanty phlegm, dry tongue with scanty fluids, thready pulse or weak feeble pulse.

Table 8　Prescriptions for Convalescent Cases with Syndrome of
Dual Deficiency of Qi and Yin

Master Prescription	Concomitant Symptom	Additive Prescription
Shengmaiyin (Pulse-Invigorating) Oral Liquid (Annex 1-28), or Baihe Gujin Wan (Lily Metal-Securing Pill) (Annex 1-21)	Poor appetite	Jianwei Xiaoshi Pian (Stomach-Strengthening Food-Digesting Tablet) (Annex 1-45)

7.1.3 Syndrome of Phlegm Coagulation and Blood Stasis(Table 9)

Clinical manifestations: Oppression in chest, suffocation, dyspnea with movement, paroxysmal dry cough, choking cough, or coughing a small amount of white phlegm, light dark tongue, thin white tongue coating or slimy coating, deep wiry pulse or unsmooth pulse.

Chest CT shows obvious signs of pulmonary interstitial lesions.

Table 9   Prescriptions for Convalescent Cases with Syndromes of
Phlegm Coagulation and Blood Stasis

Master Prescription	Concomitant Symptom	Additive Prescription
Guizhi Fuling Wan (Cinnamon-Twig Poria Pill) (Annex 1-44) or Wenfei Huaxian (Lung-Warming Fibre-Transforming) Granule.	Poor appetite	Jianwei Xiaoshi Pian (Stomach-Strengthening Food-Digesting Tablet) (Annex 1-45)
	Obvious Qi deficiency syndromes, such as dyspnea with movement, fatigue, laziness to speak	Buzhong Yiqi Wan/San (Middle-Supplementing Qi-Enriching Pill/Tea) (Annex 1-41)
	Yin deficiency syndromes, such as dry mouth, dry throat and scanty tongue coating	Shengmaiyin (Pulse-Invigorating) Oral Liquid (Annex 1-28)
	Obvious cough	Tongxuan Lifei Wan (Lung-Ventilating-Dredging-Rectifying Pill) (Annex 1-14, 1-15)

7.2 Application of Appropriate TCM Techniques

7.2.1 Acupuncture and Moxibustion Therapy

Operation method and frequency: If filiform needle is used for treatment, retain the needle for 25- 30 minutes each time for the acupuncture reinforcing purpose, once per day or once every other day. If electric needle or transcutaneous acupoint electrical stimulation is adopted, select the low frequency of 2 Hz and an electric current strength of 10-20 mA and retain the needle for 15-20 minutes each time, once per day or once every other day. Or acupoint moxibustion is applied for stimulation, once in the morning and once in the evening, 15-20 minutes each time.

[Basic Selected Acupoints] Dazhui (GV14), Zusanli (ST36), Feishu (BL13), Geshu(BL17)

(1) Syndrome of Lung and Spleen Qi Deficiency

[Selected Acupoints] Taiyuan (LU9), Danzhong (CV17), Qihai (CV6), Guanyuan (CV4).

For the case with profuse phlegm, add Fenglong (ST40), and Taibai (SP3); for aversion to cold, apply additionally moxibustion on Fengmen (BL12); for abdominal distension and loose stool, add Tianshu (ST25).

(2) Syndrome of Lung and Stomach Yin Deficiency

[Selected Acupoints] Taiyuan (LU9), Gaohuang (BL43), Taixi (KI3), and Sanyinjiao (SP6).

For the case with hemoptysis, add Kongzui (LU6); for gastric stuffiness, add Zhongwan (CV12); for constipation, add Tianshu (ST25).

(3) Syndrome of Dual Deficiency of Qi and Yin, with Residual Pathogens

[Selected Acupoints] Shenshu (BL23), Yuji (LU10), Taiyuan (LU9), Taixi (KI3), and Sanyinjiao (SP6).

For those with severe asthma, add Dingchuan (EX-B1); for insomnia, add Neiguan (PC6) and Shenmen (HT7).

7.2.2 Auricular Acupuncture Therapy

[Selected Acupoints] Lung Meridian, Pingchuan (antiasthmatic point), Shenmen on ear, Large Intestine Meridian, Endocrine Point, etc.

[Auricular application method] Perform auricular acupoint application therapy with seeds of Wangbuliuxing (Semen Vaccariae), gently press with fingers for 1-2 minutes every day, and renew it every three days.

[Contraindications] It is not indicated for use in patients with skin ulceration, skin allergy or scar constitution.

7.2.3 Acupoint Application Therapy

Chinese herbs such as Baijiezi (Semen Sinapis), Xixin (Herba Asari), Chuanxiong (Rhizoma Chuanxiong), Cangzhu (Rhizoma Atractylodis), etc., are ground into fine powder and made into medicinal cake for application.

[Selected Acupoints] Feishu (BL13), Dingchuan (EX-B1), Gaohuang (BL43), Danzhong (CV17), Fenglong (ST40), etc.

[Frequency] Once a day, 4-6 hours each time.

[Contraindications] It is not indicated for use in pregnant women, and the patients with hemoptysis, skin ulceration, skin allergy and scar constitution.

7.2.4 Moxibustion

Perform circling moxibustion with moxa stick about 1.5-3cm away from the skin. Make clockwise or anticlockwise circling movement along the bladder meridian from Fengmen (BL12) to Geshu (BL17). The duration of treatment is about 20 minutes, once every other day.

8. Precautions after Quarantine and Discharge from Hospital

8.1 Discharge Standards

8.1.1 The body temperature returns to normal for more than 3 days.

8.1.2 Significant improvement in respiratory symptoms.

8.1.3 Chest radiography shows significant improvement in acute exudative lesions.

8.1.4 Negative results of nucleic acid tests of sputum samples, nasopharyngeal swabs and other respiratory specimens for twice in a row (samplings at an interval of at least 24 hours).

Those who meet the standards above can be discharged.

8.2 Precautions after Discharge from Hospital

8.2.1 The designated hospitals should contact the community-level medical and health care institutions of the places where the patients live, share medical records, and promptly send the discharged patients' information to the competent authorities or residential committees and community-level medical and health care institutions of the places where the patients live.

8.2.2 After the patient is discharged from the hospital, it is recommended to continue the quarantine and monitor health for 14 days, and the patient should wear a mask, live in a well-ventilated single room if conditions permit, reduce close contact with family members, dine with separate plates, practice good hand hygiene and avoid going out.

8.2.3 It is recommended to make follow-up visits to the hospital in the 2nd and 4th week after discharge.

Annex 1

Standards for Prescriptions and Prescription Preparations

1. **Kuangfu Zhengqi San (Healthy-Qi-Supporting Tea)**

Origin: This prescription was worked out by Professor Liu Jingyuan (national famous veteran TCM doctor from Beijing University of Chinese Medicine) based on combination and modification of three classic prescriptions: Shengmai San (Pulse-Invigorating Tea) recorded in the *Revelation of Medicine* by Zhang Yuansu in Jin Dynasty (1127AD-1279AD), Yupingfeng San (Jade Screen Tea) recorded in the *Danxi's Experiential Therapy* in Yuan Dynasty (1347AD), and Huoxiang Zhengqi San (Agastache Qi-Rectifying Tea) recorded in the *Formulary of the Bureau of Taiping People's Welfare Pharmacy* by Chen Shiwen *et al.* in Song Dynasty.

Components: Guanghuoxiang (Herba Pogostemonis), Zisuye (Folium Perillae), Baizhi (Radix Angelicae Dahuricae), Maidong (Ophiopogonis Radix), Fangfeng (Radix Saposhnikoviae), Huangqi (Radix Astragali), Dangshen (Codonopsis Radix), Wuweizi (Fructus Schisandrae), Baizhu (Rhizoma Atractylodis Macrocephalae), Beishashen (Radix Glehniae), Shihu (Herba Dendrobii), Tianyeju (Folium Steviae Rebaudinae).

Actions: Tonify both Qi and Yin, enhance immunity, and used for uninfected population.

2. **Yupingfeng (Jade Screen) Oral Liquid**

Origin: This prescription originates from Yupingfeng San (Jade Screen Tea) documented in the *Danxi's Experiential*

Therapy in Yuan Dynasty (1347AD).

Standard source: *Chinese Pharmacopoeia* (2020, Volume I, P_{781}).

Components: Huangqi (Radix Astragali), Fangfeng (Radix Saposhnikoviae), and Fuchao Baizhu (Rhizoma Atractylodis Macrocephalae) (fried with wheat bran).

Actions: Enrich Qi, secure superficial and arrest sweating.

3. Huoxiang Zhengqi Shui (Agastache Qi-Rectifying Oral Liquid)

Origin: This prescription originates from the *Formulary of the Bureau of Taiping People's Welfare Pharmacy* by Chen Shiwen *et al.* in Song Dynasty (1151AD).

Standard source: *Chinese Pharmacopoeia* (2020 Volume I, $P_{1,881}$).

Components: Cangzhu (Rhizoma Atractylodis), Chenpi (Pericarpium Citri Reticulatae), Houpo (Cortex Magnoliae Officinalis) (processed with ginger), Baizhi (Radix Angelicae Dahuricae), Fuling (Poria), Dafupi (Pericarpium Arecae), Shengbanxia (Rhizoma Pinelliae), Gancao (Radix Glycyrrhizae) Extract, Guanghuoxiang (Herba Pogostemonis) Oil and Zisuye (Folium Perillae) Oil.

Actions: Release superficial and resolve dampness; regulate Qi and harmonize the middle.

4. Huoxiang Zhengqi Wan (Agastache Qi-Rectifying Pill, big honeyed pills)

Origin: This prescription originates from the *Formulary of the Bureau of Taiping People's Welfare Pharmacy* by Chen

Shiwen *et al.* in Song Dynasty (1151AD).

Standard source: *Compilation of National Chinese Patent Medicine Standard of the PRC: Lung System of Internal Medicine* (Volume 1, P_{455}).

Components: Cangzhu (Rhizoma Atractylodis), Chenpi (Pericarpium Citri Reticulatae), Houpo (Cortex Magnoliae Officinalis) (processed with ginger), Baizhi (Radix Angelicae Dahuricae), Fuling (Poria), Dafupi (Pericarpium Arecae), Banxia (Rhizoma Pinelliae) (processed with ginger), Gancao (Radix Glycyrrhizae), Guanghuoxiang (Herba Pogostemonis) and Zisuye (Folium Perillae).

Actions: Release superficial and abate fever; harmonize the middle and regulate Qi.

5. Huoxiang Zhengqi Wan (Agastache Qi-Rectifying Pills, water-honeyed pills)

Origin: This prescription originates from the *Formulary of the Bureau of Taiping People's Welfare Pharmacy* by Chen Shiwen *et al.* in Song Dynasty (1151AD).

Standard source: *Compilation of National Chinese Patent Medicine Standard of the PRC: Lung System of Internal Medicine* (Volume 1, P_{455}).

Components: Cangzhu (Rhizoma Atractylodis), Chenpi (Pericarpium Citri Reticulatae), Houpo (Cortex Magnoliae Officinalis) (processed with ginger), Baizhi (Radix Angelicae Dahuricae), Fuling (Poria), Dafupi (Pericarpium Arecae), Banxia (Rhizoma Pinelliae) (processed with ginger), Gancao (Radix Glycyrrhizae), Guanghuoxiang (Herba Pogostemonis) and Zisuye (Folium Perillae).

Actions: Release superficial and abate fever; harmonize the middle and regulate Qi.

6. Huoxiang Zhengqi Wan (Agastache Qi-Rectifying Pill, water-bindered pill)

Origin: This prescription originates from the *Formulary of the Bureau of Taiping People's Welfare Pharmacy* by Chen Shiwen *et al.* in Song Dynasty (1151 AD).

Standard source: *Compilation of National Chinese Patent Medicine Standard of the PRC: Lung System of Internal Medicine* (Volume 1, P$_{455}$).

Components: Cangzhu (Rhizoma Atractylodis), Chenpi (Pericarpium Citri Reticulatae), Houpo (Cortex Magnoliae Officinalis) (processed with ginger), Baizhi (Radix Angelicae Dahuricae), Fuling (Poria), Dafupi (Pericarpium Arecae), Banxia (Rhizoma Pinelliae) (processed with ginger), Gancao (Radix Glycyrrhizae), Guanghuoxiang (Herba Pogostemonis) and Zisuye (Folium Perillae).

Actions: Release superficial and abate fever; harmonize the middle and regulate Qi.

7. Xiaochaihu (Minor Bupleurum) Granule

Origin: This prescription originates from the *Treatise on Cold Damage and Miscellaneous Diseases* in Han Dynasty (219 AD).

Standard source: *Chinese Pharmacopoeia* (2020 Volume I, P_{605}).

Components: Chaihu (Radix Bupleuri), Huangqin (Radix Scutellariae), Banxia (Rhizoma Pinelliae) (processed with ginger), Dangshen (Radix Codonopsis), Shengjiang (Rhizoma Zingiberis Recens), Gancao (Radix Glycyrrhizae), and Dazao (Fructus Jujubae).

Actions: Release superficial and dissipate fever; soothe liver and harmonize stomach.

8. Qingre Bawei (Heat-Clearing Eight-Ingredients) Capsule

Origin: This prescription, as a traditional Mongolian medicine formula, originates from *The Four Medical Tantras* in the 8th century AD. And the eight ingredients in the formula are also referred to as eight Classical medicines.

Standard source: National Drug Standards of China State Food and Drug Administration ZZ-8404-1.

Components: Tanxiang (Lignum Santali Albi), Shigao (Gypsum Fibrosum), Honghua (Flos Carthami), Kudiding (Herba Corydalis Bungeanae), Qumai (Herba Dianthi), Huhuanglian (Rhizoma Picrorrhizae), Maidong (Radix Ophiopogonis) and Rengong Niuhuang (Calculus Bovis Artifactus).

Actions: Clear heat and remove toxin. Used for visceral fever, cough due to lung heat, bloody phlegm, liver-fire and hypochondriac pain.

9. **Lianhua Qingwen (Forsythia Honeysuckle Epidemic-Cleaning) Capsule**

Origin: This prescription is made by modifying Yinqiao San (Honeysuckle and Forsythia Tea), recorded in the *Detailed Analysis of Warm Diseases* by Wu Tang (also known as Wu Jutong) in Qing Dynasty (1798 AD), and Maxing Shigan Tang (Ephedra-Almond-Licorice-Gypsum Decotion), recorded in the *Treatise on Cold Damage* by Zhang Ji (also known as Zhang Zhongjing) in Han Dynasty (219 AD).

Standard source: *Chinese Pharmacopoeia* (2020, Volume I, $P_{1,014}$).

Components: Lianqiao (Fructus Forsythiae), Jinyinhua (Flos Lonicerae), Zhimahuang (Herba Ephedrae) (fried with honey), Chaokuxingren (Semen Armeniacae Amarum) (fried), Shigao (Gypsum Fibrosum), Banlangen (Radix Isatidis), Mianma Guanzhong (Rhizoma Dryopteridis Crassirhizomatis), Yuxingcao (Herba Houttuyniae), Guanghuoxiang (Herba Pogostemonis), Dahuang (Radix et Rhizoma Rhei), Hongjingtian (Herba Rhodiolae Sacrae), menthol and Gancao (Radix Glycyrrhizae).

Actions: Clear virus and remove toxin; ventilate lung and discharge heat.

10. **Lianhua Qingwen (orsythia Honeysuckle Epedemic-Cleaning) Granule**

Origin: This prescription is made by modifying Yinqiao San (Honeysuckle and Forsythia Tea), recorded in *Detailed*

Analysis of Warm Diseases by Wu Tang (also known as Wu Ju-tong) in Qing Dynasty (1798 AD), and Maxing Shigan Tang (Ephedra-Almond-Licorice-Gypsum Decotion), recorded in *Treatise on Cold Damage* by Zhang Ji (also known as Zhang Zhong-jing) in Han Dynasty (219 AD).

Standard source: *Chinese Pharmacopoeia* (2020, Volume I, $P_{1,015}$).

Components: Lianqiao (Fructus Forsythiae), Jinyinhua (Flos Lonicerae), Zhimahuang (Herba Ephedrae) (fried with honey), Chaokuxingren (Semen Armeniacae Amarum) (fried), Shigao (Gypsum Fibrosum), Banlangen (Radix Isatidis), Mianma Guanzhong (Rhizoma Dryopteridis Crassirhizomatis), Yuxingcao (Herba Houttuyniae), Guanghuoxiang (Herba Pogostemonis), Dahuang (Radix et Rhizoma Rhei), Hongjingtian (Herba Rhodiolae Sacrae), menthol and Gancao (Radix Glycyrrhizae).

Actions: Clear virus and remove toxin; ventilate lung and discharge heat.

11. Jinhua Qinggan (Honeysuckle Cold-Clearing) Granule

Origin: This prescription originates from Jinhua Qinggan Formula (Honeysuckle Cold-Clearing Formula) which has been repeatedly screened and optimized on the basis of the experts' clinical experience and over one hundred ancient prescriptions in TCM classics such as the *Treatise on Cold Damage* by Zhang Ji (i.e. Zhang Zhongjing) in Han Dynasty (219 BC), the *On Pestilence* by Wu Youke in Ming Dynasty (1641AD) and the *Detailed Analysis of Warm Diseases* by Wu Tang (i.e. Wu Jutong) in Qing Dynasty (1798AD).

Standard source: Standards of China State Food and Drug Administration YBZ00392016.

Components: Jinyinhua (Flos Lonicerae), Shigao (Gypsum Fibrosum), Mimahuang (Herba Ephedrae) (fried with honey), Chaokuxingren (Semen Armeniacae Amarum) (fried), Huangqin (Radix Scutellariae), Lianqiao (Fructus Forsythiae), Zhebeimu (Bulbus Fritillariae Thunbergii), Zhimu (Rhizoma Anemarrhenae), Niubangzi (Fructus Arctii), Qinghao (Herba Artemisiae Annuae), Bohe (Herba Menthae) and Gancao (Radix Glycyrrhizae).

Actions: Disperse wind and ventilate lung; clear heat and remove toxin.

12. Jiuwei Qianghuo Wan (Nine-Ingredients Notopterygium Pill)

Origin: This prescription was created by renowned doctor Zhang Yuansu in Jin Dynasty and recorded in the *Medical Book for Difficult Problems* by Wang Haogu, a doctor in Yuan Dynasty (1279-1368AD) who studied medicine under Li Gao, a disciple of Zhang Yuansu.

Standard source: *Chinese Pharmacopoeia* (2020, Volume I, P$_{501}$).

Components: Qianghuo (Rhizoma et Radix Notopterygii), Fangfeng (Radix Saposhnikoviae), Cangzhu (Rhizoma Atractylodis), Xixin (Herba Asari), Chuanxiong

(Rhizoma Chuanxiong), Baizhi (Radix Angelicae Dahuricae), Huangqin (Radix Scutellariae), Gancao (Radix Glycyrrhizae) and Dihuang (Radix Rehmanniae).

Actions: Disperse wind and release superficial; dissipate cold and remove dampness.

13. Chuanxiong Chatiao (Ligusticum Tea-Making) Granule

Origin: This prescription originates from Chuanxiong Chatiao San (Ligusticum Tea-Making Tea) in the *Formulary of the Bureau of Taiping People's Welfare Pharmacy* in Song Dynasty (1078-1085AD).

Standard source: *Chinese Pharmacopoeia* (2020 Volume I, P_{546}).

Components: Chuanxiong (Rhizoma Chuanxiong), Baizhi (Radix Angelicae Dahuricae), Qianghuo (Rhizoma et Radix Notopterygii), Xixin (Herba Asari), Fangfeng (Radix Saposhnikoviae), Jingjie (Herba Schizonepetae), Bohe (Herba Menthae) and Gancao (Radix Glycyrrhizae).

Actions: Disperse wind and relieve pain.

14. Tongxuan Lifei Wan (Lung-Ventilating-Dredging-Rectifying Pill, big honeyed pills)

Origin: This prescription, originally a modification of Zisu Yin (Perillae Decoction), comes from the *Criterion for Pattern Identification and Treatment* by Wang Kentang in Ming Dynasty (1602AD).

Standard source: *Chinese Pharmacopoeia* (2020, Volume I, $P_{1,571}$) .

Components: Zisuye (Folium Perillae), Qianhu (Radix Peucedani),

Jiegeng (Radix Platycodi), Kuxingren (Semen Armeniacae Amarum), Mahuang (Herba Ephedrae), Gancao (Radix Glycyrrhizae), Chenpi (Pericarpium Citri Reticulatae), Banxia (Rhizoma Pinelliae) (processed), Fuling (Poria), Zhike (Fructus Aurantii) (fried) and Huangqin (Radix Scutellariae).

Actions: Release superficial and dissipate cold; ventilate lung and stop cough.

15. Tongxuan Lifei Wan (Lung-Ventilating-Dredging-Rectifying Pill, water-honeyed pills)

Origin: This prescription, originally a modification of Zisu Yin (Perillae Decoction), comes from the *Criterion for Pattern Identification and Treatment* by Wang Kentang in Ming Dynasty (1602AD).

Standard source: *Chinese Pharmacopoeia* (2020, Volume I, $P_{1,571}$).

Components: Zisuye (Folium Perillae), Qianhu (Radix Peucedani), Jiegeng (Radix Platycodi), Kuxingren (Semen Armeniacae Amarum), Mahuang (Herba Ephedrae), Gancao (Radix Glycyrrhizae), Chenpi (Pericarpium Citri Reticulatae), Banxia (Rhizoma Pinelliae) (processed), Fuling (Poria), Zhike (Fructus Aurantii) (fried), and Huangqin (Radix Scutellariae).

Actions: Release superficial and dissipate cold; ventilate lung and stop cough.

16. **Guilong Kechuanning (Cinnamon-Twig Dragon-Bone Cough-Panting-Calming) Tablet**

Origin: This prescription originates from the *Synopsis of the Golden Chamber* by Zhang Zhongjing in Eastern Han Dynasty (206 AD).

Standard source: *Chinese Pharmacopoeia* (2020, Volume I, $P_{1,431}$).

Components: Guizhi (Ramulus Cinnamomi), Longgu (Os Draconis), Baishao (Radix Paeoniae Alba), Shengjiang (Rhizoma Zingiberis Recens), Dazao (Fructus Jujubae), Zhigancao (Radix Glycyrrhizae) (fried with honey), Muli (Concha Ostreae), Huanglian (Rhizoma Coptidis), Fabanxia (Rhizoma Pinelliae) (processed), Gualoupi (Pericarpium Trichosanthis), and Chaokuxingren (Semen Armeniacae Amarum) (fried).

Actions: Stop cough and resolve phlegm; descend Qi and relieve panting.

17. **Xianzhuli (Fresh Bamboo Juice) Oral Liquid**

Origin: This prescription originates from the *Collective Commentaries on Classics of Materia Medica* (about before 480-498 AD).

Standard source: *China Health Ministry Drug Standards: Traditional Chinese Medicinals* (1992, Volume 1, P_{99}), Single-Page Standards of China State Food and Drug Administration (2004).

Components: The liquid got by heating the fresh stalk of Phyllostachys glauca McClure, Phyllostachysnuda McClure or other plants of the same genus.

Actions: Clear heat and resolve phlegm.

18. Yingqiao Jiedu Wan (Honeysuckle Forsythia Toxin-Resolving Pill)

Origin: This prescription originates from the *Detailed Analysis of Warm Diseases* by Wu Tang in Qing Dynasty (1798 AD).

Standard source: *China Health Ministry Drug Standards: TCM Prescription Preparation* (Volume 19, P_{200}).

Components: Jinyinhua (Flos Lonicerae), Lianqiao (Fructus Forsythiae), Bohe (Herba Menthae), Jingjie (Herba Schizonepetae), Dandouchi (Semen Sojae Preparatum), Niubangzi (Fructus Arctii) (fried), Jiegeng (Radix Platycodi), Danzhuye (Herba Lophatheri) and Gancao (Radix Glycyrrhizae).

Actions: Disperse wind and release superficial; clear heat and remove toxin.

19. Sanhuang Pian (Scutellaria Coptis Phellodendron Tablet)

Origin: This prescription, composed of Dahuang (Radix et Rhizoma Rhei), Huangqin (Radix Scutellariae) and Huanglian (Rhizoma Coptidis) and named "Sanhuang", originates from Xiexin Tang (Heart-Draining Decoction) in the *Synopsis of the Golden Chamber* by Zhang Zhongjing in Eastern Han Dynasty (206 AD), and endured for thousands of years.

Standard source: *Chinese Pharmacopoeia* (2020, Volume I, P_{517}).

Components: Dahuang (Radix et Rhizoma Rhei), Berberine Hydrochloride, and Huangqin (Radix Scutellariae) Extract.

Actions: Clear heat and remove toxin; reduce fire and promote
defecation.

20. Baihe Gujin Wan (Lily Metal-Securing Pill, concentrated pills)

Origin: This medicine is concentrated from Baihe Guijin Wan,
which originates from the *Collected Exegesis of Prescriptions*
by Wang Ang in Qing Dynasty (1682 AD)

Standard source: *Chinese Pharmacopoeia* (2020, Volume I, P_{880}) .

Components: Baihe (Bulbus Lilii), Dihuang (Radix Rehmanniae),
Shudihuang (Radix Rehmanniae) (processed), Maidong
(Radix Ophiopogonis), Xuanshen (Radix Scrophulariae),
Chuanbeimu (Bulbus Frityllariae Cirrhosae), Danggui
(Radix Angelicae Sinensis), Baishao (Radix Paeoniae
Alba), Jiegeng (Radix Platycodi) and Gancao (Radix
Glycyrrhizae).

Actions: Nourish Yin and moisten lung; resolve phlegm and stop
cough.

21. Baihe Gujin Wan (Lily Metal-Securing Pill)

Origin: This prescription originates from the *Collected Exegesis of
Prescriptions* by Wang Ang in Qing Dynasty (1682 AD).

Standard source: *Chinese Pharmacopoeia* (2020, Volume I, P_{879}).

Components: Baihe (Bulbus Lilii), Dihuang (Radix Rehmanniae),
Shudihuang (Radix Rehmanniae)(processed), Maidong
(Radix Ophiopogonis), Xuanshen (Radix Scrophulariae)
Chuanbeimu (Bulbus Frityllariae Cirrhosae), Danggui

(Radix Angelicae Sinensis), Baishao (Radix Paeoniae Alba), Jiegeng (Radix Platycodi) and Gancao (Radix Glycyrrhizae).

Actions: Nourish Yin and moisten lung; resolve phlegm and stop cough.

22. Anshen Buxin Liuwei Wan (Spirit-Calming Heart-Tonifying Six-Ingredients Pill)

Origin: This prescription originates from *The Four Medical Entrant* by Yutuo Ningma · Yundan Gongbu in the 8th century.

Standard source: National Drug Standards of China State Food and Drug Administration ZZ-8324-1.

Components: Niuxin (Cor Bovis seu Bubali), Muxiang (Radix Aucklandiae), Fengxiangzhi (Resina Liquidambaris), Dingxiang (Flos Caryophylli), Roudoukou (Semen Myristicae) and Guangzao (Fructus Choerospondiatis).

Actions: Remove "Hè yī disease" in Mongolian medicine; tranquilize mind; treat palpitation and shortness of breath.

23. Jiedu Yiqi San (Toxin-Resolving Qi-Enriching Tea)

Origin: This prescription was created by Professor Liu Jingyuan (national famous veteran TCM doctor from Beijing University of Chinese Medicine) combining and modifying Zhisou San (Cough-Stopping Tea), Yupingfeng San (Jade Screen Tea) recorded in the *Danxi's Experiential Therapy* in Yuan Dynasty (1347AD), and Huoxiang

Zhengqi San (Agastache Qi-Rectifying Tea) recorded in the *Formulary of the Bureau of Taiping People's Welfare Pharmacy* by Chen Shiwen *et al.* in Song Dynasty.

Components: Guanghuoxiang (Herba Pogostemonis), Zisuye (Folium Perillae), Baizhi (Radix Angelicae Dahuricae), Dangshen (Radix Codonopsis), Qingbanxia (Rhizoma Pinelliae) (processed with alum), Huangqi (Radix Astragali), Beishashen (Radix Glehniae), Maidong (Radix Ophiopogonis), Fangfeng (Radix Saposhnikoviae), Zhebeimu (Bulbus Fritillariae Thunbergii), Jinyinhua (Flos Lonicerae), Huangqin (Radix Scutellariae), Xiebai (Bulbus Allii Macrostemi), Xingren (Semen Armeniacae Amarum), Gualoupi (Pericarpium Trichosanthis), Zhikuandonghua (Flos Farfarae) (fried with honey), Zhiziwan (Radix Asteris) (fried with honey), Sangbaipi (Cortex Mori), Sangye (Folium Mori), Shihu (Herba Dendrobii), and Tianyeju (Folium Steviae Rebaudinae).

Actions: Cold and warm medicinals are combined together to eliminate pathogens and strengthen healthy Qi. Qi-enriching and Yin-nourishing medicinals with mild property are prescribed simultaneously. It is indicated for treatment of suspected cases, mild and common syndromes, and can also serve as a complementary therapy to western medicine for severe cases.

24. **Huashi Baidu (Dampness-Resolving Toxin-Defeating) Granule**

Origin: *Diagnosis and Treatment Protocol for COVID-19 (The 7th Trial Edition)* from National Health Commission of the PRC.

Components: Mahuang (Herba Ephedrae), Xingren (Semen Armeniacae Amarum), Shigao (Gypsum Fibrosum), Gancao (Radix Glycyrrhizae), Guanghuoxiang (Herba Pogostemonis), Houpo (Cortex Magnoliae Officinalis), Cangzhu (Rhizoma Atractylodis), Caoguo (Fructus Tsaoko), Fabanxia (Rhizoma Pinelliae Preparatum), Fuling (Poria), Chishao (Radix Paeoniae Rubra), Dahuang (Radix et Rhizoma Rhei), Huangqi (Radix Astragali seu Hedysari) and Tinglizi (Semen Descurainiae).

Actions: Resolve dampness and expel filth; ventilate lung and unblock organs; activate blood and remove toxin.

25. **Niuhuang Qingxin Wan (Bezoar Heart-Clearing Pill)**

Origin: This prescription originates from the *Formulary of the Bureau of Taiping People's Welfare Pharmacy* by Chen Shiwen *et al.* in Song Dynasty (1151 AD).

Standard source: *Chinese Pharmacopoeia* (2020, Volume I, P$_{690}$).

Components: Niuhuang (Calculus Bovis), Danggui (Radix Angelicae Sinensis), Chuanxiong (Rhizoma Chuanxiong), Gancao (Radix Glycyrrhizae), Shaoyao (Rhizoma Dioscoreae), Huangqin (Radix Scutellariae), Kuxingren (Semen Armeniacae Amarum) (fried), Dadou Huangjuan (Semen

Glycines Siccus), Dazao (Fructus Jujubae), Baizhu (Rhizoma Atractylodis Macrocephalae) (fried), Fuling (Poria), Jiegeng (Radix Platycodi), Fangfeng (Radix Saposhnikoviae), Chaihu (Radix Bupleuri), Ejiao (Colla Corii Asini), Ganjiang (Rhizoma Zingiberis), Baishao (Radix Paeoniae Alba), Renshen (Radix Ginseng), Liushenqu (Medicated Leaven)(fried), Rougui (Cortex Cinnamomi), Maidong (Radix Ophiopogonis), Bailian (Radix Ampelopsis), Puhuang (Pollen Typhae) (fried), Rengong Shexiang (Moschus Artifactus), Bingpian (Borneolum Syntheticum), Shuiniujiao Nongsuofen (Pulvis Cornus Bubali Concentratus), Lingyangjiao (Cornu Saigae Tataricae), Zhusha (Cinnabaris) and Xionghuang (Realgar).

Actions: Clear heat and remove toxin; open orifices and tranquilize mind.

26. Angong Niuhuang Wan (Heart-Calming Bezoar Pill)

Origin: This prescription originates from Line 16 of *Chapter Upper Energizer* in the *Detailed Analysis of Warm Diseases* by Wu Jutong in Qing Dynasty.

Standard source: *Chinese Pharmacopoeia* (2020, Volume I, P_{930}), and its corrected and supplemented version (P95).

Components: Niuhuang (Calculus Bovis), Shuiniujiao Nongsuofen (Pulvis Cornus Bubali Concentratus), Rengong Shexiang (Moschus Artifactus), Zhenzhu (Margarita), Zhusha (Cinnabaris), Xionghuang (Realgar), Huanglian

(Rhizoma Coptidis), Huangqin (Radix Scutellariae), Zhizi (Fructus Gardeniae), Yujin (Radix Curcumae) and Bingpian (Borneolum Syntheticum).

Actions: Clear heat and remove toxin; calm fright and open orifices.

27. **Pianzaihuang (made of Bezoar, musk, etc.)**

Origin: This prescription was originally confidential among the imperial physicians in Ming Dynasty. But all the records, including the secret prescription among the imperial physicians, were lost during the Ming Dynasty turmoil. The only thing that can be known about it was the Li Shizhen's records of Sanqi (Radix Notoginseng) in the *Compendium of Materia Medica*. The book recorded that Sanqi (Radix Notoginseng), both rare and expensive, was produced in the southern mountains, and it was introduced to royal court and made into Pianzaihuang through special technique, which was later designated as a royal confidential prescription. The technology was incorporated into Zhangzhou Pharmaceutical Factory in 1956.

Standard source: *Chinese Pharmacopoeia* (2020, Volume I, P_{703}).

Components: Niuhuang (Calculus Bovis), Shexiang (Moschus), Sanqi (Radix Notoginseng), Shedan (Fel Serpentis), etc.

Actions: Clear heat and remove toxin; cool blood and resolve blood stasis; disperse swelling and stop pain.

28.   Shengmaiyin (Pulse-Invigorating) Oral Liquid

Origin:
This prescription, as one of the tonifying prescriptions, originates from the *Revelation of Medicine* by Zhang Yuansu in Jin Dynasty (1127-1279AD).

Standard source:
China Health Ministry Drug Standards: TCM Prescription Preparation (Volume 12, P_{39}).

Components:
Dangshen (Radix Codonopsis), Maidong (Radix Ophiopogonis) and Wuweizi (Fructus Schisandrae).

Actions:
Enrich Qi and invigorate pulse; nourish Yin and promote fluid.

29.   Yunnan Baiyao (mainly made of panax pseudo-ginseng of Yunnan Province)

Origin:
This prescription, previously known as Huanzhang's Baibaodan, was developed by Qu Huanzhang in 1902.

Standard source:
Chinese Pharmacopoeia (2020, Volume I, P_{636}).

Components:
Sanqi (Radix Notoginseng), Chonglou (Rhizoma Paridis), etc.

Actions:
Clear heat and remove toxin; calm fright and open orifices.

30.   Xiyanping (Happiness Inflammation-Deleting) Injection

Origin:
Drug Standards of Jiangxi Province (1982).

Standard source:
Compilation of National Chinese Patent Medicine Standard of the PRC: Lung System of Internal Medicine (Volume 1, P455), Revised Standard WS-10863(ZD-0863)-2002-2011Z.

Components: Andrographolide Sulfonate.

Actions: Clear heat and remove toxin; stop cough and check dysentery.

31. Tanreqing (Phlegm-Heat-Clearing) Injection

Origin: This prescription was created by adding heat-clearing medicinals such as Shanyangjiao (Cornu Caprinus) and Xiongdan (Fel Ursi) Powder into Shuanghuanglian (combination of Honeysuckle, Scutellariae and Forsythia), which is composed on the basis of Dalianqiao Tang (Great Forsythia Decoction), recorded in the *Guide for Children's Diseases* (Volume V) by Yang Shiying (also known as Yang Renzhai) in Song Dynasty (1206 AD) and Yinqiao San (Honeysuckle and Forsythia Tea), recorded in the *Detailed Analysis of Warm Diseases* by Wu Tang (also known as Wu Jutong) in Qing Dynasty (1798 AD).

Standard source: New Medicine Regularization Standard (Volume 75, P_8) and Standards of China State Food and Drug Administration YBZ00912003-2007Z-2009.

Components: Huangqin (Radix Scutellariae), Xiongdan (Fel Ursi) Powder, Shanyangjiao (Cornu Caprinus), Jinyinhua (Flos Lonicerae), and Lianqiao (Fructus Forsythiae).

Actions: Clear heat, resolve phlegm, and remove toxin.

32. Xingnaojing (Brain-Waking-Calming) Injection

Origin: This prescription originates from *China Health Ministry Drug Standards: TCM Prescription Preparation* (Volume 17) in modern times (1998). It is a reduced version of Angong Niuhuang Wan (Heart-Calming Bezoar Pill) recorded in the *Detailed Analysis of Warm Diseases* in Qing Dynasty (1798 AD)

Standard source: *China Health Ministry Drug Standards: TCM Prescription Preparation* (Volume 17, P278).

Components: Rengong Shexiang (Moschus Artifactus), Yujin (Radix Curcumae), Bingpian (Borneolum Syntheticum) and Zhizi (Fructus Gardeniae).

Actions: Clear heat and remove toxin; cool blood and activate blood; open orifices and awaken brain.

33. Xuebijing (Blood-Must-Be-Clear) Injection

Origin: Standard of State Food and Drug Administration Standard (2012). This injection was refined from Xuefu Zhuyu Tang (Decoction for Removing Blood Stasis in the Chest) by Professor Wang Jinda, the founder of Integrated Traditional Chinese and Western Emergency Medicine. Xuefu Zhuyu Tang originates from the *Correction on Errors in Medical Works* published in 1830.

Standard source: China YBZ01242004-2010Z-2012.

Components: Honghua (Flos Carthami), Chishao (Radix Paeoniae Rubra), Chuanxiong (Rhizoma Chuanxiong), Danshen (Radix Salviae Miltiorrhizae) and Danggui (Radix Angelicae Sinensis).

Actions: Resolve blood stasis and remove toxin.

34.   **Shenmai (Ginseng Ophiopogon) Injection**

Origin: This prescription was prepared from Hongshen (Radix Ginseng Destillata) and Maidong (Radix Ophiopogonis), whose ingredients originate from Shengmaiyin (Pulse-Invigorating) Oral Liquid recorded in the *On Syndrome Cause Pulse and Treatment* published in 1706.

Standard source: *China Health Ministry Drug Standards: TCM Prescription Preparation* (Volume 18, P_{170}), Revised Standard ZGB2010-7, and Revised Standard 2011B011.

Components: Hongshen (Radix Ginseng Destillata) and Maidong (Radix Ophiopogonis).

Actions: Enrich Qi and stop collapse; nourish Yin and promote fluid production; invigorate pulse.

35.   **Shenfu (Ginseng Aconite) Injection**

Origin: This prescription originates from Shenfu Tang (Ginseng Aconite Decoction) recorded in the *Mr. Yan's Formulas to Aid the Living* by Yan Yonghe in Southern Song Dynasty (1253 AD).

Standard source: Standards for Chinese medicinal issued by Ministries in China (Volume 18), Z18-167; Standard NO: WS3-B-3427-98.

Components: Extracts from Hongshen (Radix Ginseng Destillata) and Heifupian (Radix Aconiti Lateralis Preparata) (in slices).

Actions: Recuperate Yang and prevent collapse; enrich Qi and stop collapse.

36. Chaihu (Bupleurum) Injection

Origin: This injection is a saturated aqueous solution prepared from Bupleurum chinense DC. or Bupleurum scorzonerifolium Willd. by steam distillation, seen in the *China Health Ministry Drug Standards: TCM Prescription Preparation* (Volume 17).

Standard source: *China Health Ministry Drug Standards: TCM Prescription Preparation* (Volume 17, P_{211}), *Compilation of National Chinese Patent Medicine Standard of the PRC: Lung System of Internal Medicine* (Volume 1, P_{416}), and SFDA Standard (2011).

Components: Beichaihu (Radix Bupleuri).

Actions: Clear heat and release superficial.

37. Mengtuoshi San (Smectite Tea)

Origin: A modern prescription, composed by only one mineral medicine.

Standard source: *Chinese Pharmacopoeia* (2020, Volume II, $P_{1,723}$).

Components: Mengtuoshi (Smectite).

Actions: Check diarrhea.

38. Suhexiang Wan (Liquidambar Pill)

Origin: This prescription originates from the *Formulary of the Bureau of Taiping People's Welfare Pharmacy* in Song Dynasty (1151AD).

Standard source: *Chinese Pharmacopoeia* (2020, Volume I, P_{996}).

Components: Suhexiang (Styrax), Anxixiang (Benzoinum), Bingpian (Borneolum Syntheticum), Shuiniujiao Nongsuofen

(Pulvis Cornus Bubali Concentratus), Rengong Shexiang (Moschus Artifactus), Tanxiang (Lignum Santali Albi), Chenxiang (Lignum Aquilariae Resinatum), Dingxiang (Flos Caryophylli), Xiangfu (Rhizoma Cyperi), Muxiang (Radix Aucklandiae), Ruxiang (Olibanum)(processed), Biba (Fructus Piperis Longi), Baizhu (Rhizoma Atractylodis Macrocephalae), Hezirou (Fructus Chebulae) and Zhusha (Cinnabaris).

Actions: Open orifices with aromatic herbs, move Qi and stop pain.

39.   Shenling Baizhu San (Codnopsis Poria Ovate Atractylodes Tea)

Origin: This prescription originates from the *Formulary of the Bureau of Taiping People's Welfare Pharmacy* in 1078-1085 AD.

Standard source: *Chinese Pharmacopoeia* (2020, Volume I, $P_{1,223}$).

Components: Renshen (Radix Ginseng), Fuling (Poria), Baizhu (Rhizoma Atractylodis Macrocephalae) (fried), Shanyao (Rhizoma Dioscoreae), Baibiandou (Semen Lablab Album)(fried), Lianzi (Semen Nelumbinis), Yiyiren (Semen Coicis)(fried), Sharen (Fructus Amomi), Jiegeng (Radix Platycodi) and Gancao (Radix Glycyrrhizae).

Actions: Tonify spleen and stomach; enrich lung Qi.

40. **Shenling Baizhu Wan (Codnopsis Poria Ovate Atractylodes Pill)**

Origin: This prescription originates from Shenlin Baizhu San (Codnopsis Poria Ovate Atractylodes Tea) in the *Formulary of the Bureau of Taiping People's Welfare Pharmacy* in 1078-1085 AD.

Standard source: *Chinese Pharmacopoeia* (2020, Volume I, $P_{1,222}$).

Components: Renshen (Radix Ginseng), Fuling (Poria), Fuchao Baizhu (Rhizoma Atractylodis Macrocephalae) (fried with wheat bran), Shanyao (Rhizoma Dioscoreae), Chaobaibiandou (Semen Lablab Album) (fried). Lianzi (Semen Nelumbinis), Fuchao Yiyiren (Semen Coicis) (fried with wheat bran), Sharen (Fructus Amomi), Jiegeng (Radix Platycodi) and Gancao (Radix Glycyrrhizae).

Actions: Tonify spleen and stomach; enrich lung Qi.

41. **Buzhong Yiqi Wan (Middle-Supplementing Qi-Enriching Pill)**

Origin: This prescription originates from Buzhong Yiqi Tang (Middle-Supplementing Qi-Enriching Decoction) recorded in the *Treatise on Spleen and Stomach* by Li Dongyuan in Jin Dynasty (1249 AD).

Standard source: *Chinese Pharmacopoeia* (2020, Volume I, $P_{1,063}$).

Components: Zhihuangqi (Radix Astragali)(fried with honey), Dangshen (Radix Codonopsis), Zhigancao (Radix Glycyrrhizae) (fried with honey), Baizhu (Rhizoma Atractylodis Macrocephalae) (fried), Danggui (Radix Angelicae Sinensis), Shengma (Rhizoma Cimicifugae),

Chaihu (Radix Bupleuri), Chenpi (Pericarpium Citri Reticulatae), Shengjiang (Rhizoma Zingiberis Recens), and Dazao (Fructus Jujubae).

Actions: Supplement the middle and enrich Qi; elevate Yang and raise the drooping.

42. Xiangsha Liujun Wan (Cyperus Amomum Six-Gentlemen Pill)

Origin: This prescription originates from the *Collected Exegesis of Prescriptions* in 1682 AD.

Standard source: *Chinese Pharmacopoeia* (2020, Volume I, $P_{1,292}$) .

Components: Muxiang (Radix Aucklandiae), Sharen (Fructus Amomi), Dangshen (Radix Codonopsis), Baizhu (Rhizoma Atractylodis Macrocephalae) (fried), Fuling (Poria), Gancao (Radix Glycyrrhizae) (fried with honey), Chenpi (Pericarpium Citri Reticulatae) and Banxia (Rhizoma Pinelliae) (processed with ginger).

Actions: Enrich Qi, invigorate spleen, and harmonize stomach.

43. Xiaoyao Wan (Care-Free Pill)

Origin: This prescription originates from Xiaoyao San (Care-Free Tea) recorded in the *Formulary of the Bureau of Taiping People's Welfare Pharmacy* in 1078-1085 AD.

Standard source: *Chinese Pharmacopoeia* (2020, Volume I, $P_{1,461}$).

Components: Chaihu (Radix Bupleuri), Danggui (Radix Angelicae Sinensis), Baishao (Radix Paeoniae Alba), Fuchao Baizhu (Rhizoma Atractylodis Macrocephalae) (fried with wheat bran), Fuling (Poria), Gancao (Radix Glycyrrhizae) (fried with honey), Bohe (Herba Menthae) and Shengjiang (Rhizoma Zingiberis Recens).

Actions: Soothe liver and invigorate spleen; nourish blood and regulate menstruation.

44. **Guizhi Fuling Wan (Cinnamon-Twig Poria Pill)**

Origin: This prescription originates from the *Synopsis of the Golden Chamber* by Zhang Zhongjing in Eastern Han Dynasty (206 AD).

Standard source: *Chinese Pharmacopoeia* (2020, Volume I, $P_{1,439}$).

Components: Guizhi (Ramulus Cinnamomi), Fuling (Poria), Mudanpi (Cortex Moutan Radicis), Chishao (Radix Paeoniae Rubra) and Taoren (Semen Persicae).

Actions: Activate blood, resolve blood stasis, and subdue abdominal mass.

45. **Jianwei Xiaoshi Pian (Stomach-Strengthening Food-Digesting Tablet)**

Origin: This prescription originates from the *Criterion for Pattern Identification and Treatment* by Wang Kentang in Ming Dynasty (1602 AD).

Standard source: *Chinese Pharmacopoeia* (2020, Volume I, $P_{1,474}$).

Components: Taizishen (Radix Pseudostellariae), Chenpi (Pericarpium Citri Reticulatae), Shanyao (Rhizoma Dioscoreae), Chaomaiya (Fructus Hordei Germinatus) (fried) and Shanzha (Fructus Crataegi).

Actions: Strengthen stomach and promote digestion.

Annex 2

COVID-19 Clinical Syndrome Score Scale

Name: Gender: Age: Contact information:

Admission date:		Total score:		
Items	No	Mild	Medium	Severe
Fever	☐$_0$ No	☐$_3$ 37.3-38.5℃	☐$_6$ 38.6-39.5℃	☐$_9$ Above 39.5℃
Aversion to cold	☐$_0$ No	☐$_3$ Mild aversion to wind	☐$_6$ Aversion to cold, which cannot be relieved by putting on more clothes	☐$_9$ Shiver
Head and body aches	☐$_0$ No	☐$_3$ Slight head and body aches, which occur from time to time	☐$_6$ Continuous endurable head and body aches	☐$_9$ Severe unbearable head and body aches
Head and body heaviness	☐$_0$ No	☐$_3$ Slight head and body heaviness	☐$_6$ Continuous head and body heaviness, with limited movement ability	☐$_9$ Severe head and body heaviness, with no movement ability
Fatigue	☐$_0$ No	☐$_3$ Fatigue which does not affect daily work	☐$_6$ Fatigue, with limited movement ability	☐$_9$ Severe fatigue, with no willingness to move
Sweating	☐$_0$ No	☐$_3$ Occasional sweating	☐$_6$ A little bit sweating, without wetting clothes	☐$_9$ Profuse sweating
Cough	☐$_0$ No	☐$_3$ Occasional coughing	☐$_6$ Paroxysmal coughing	☐$_9$ Frequent coughing
Expectoration	☐$_0$ No	☐$_3$ Expectorating sometimes	☐$_6$ Expectorating often	☐$_9$ Expectorating frequently with abundant phlegm

Items	No	Mild	Medium	Severe
Nasal obstruction	☐0 No	☐3 Slight nasal obstruction	Nasal obstruction, runny nose, or yellow mucus	☐9 Continuous nasal obstruction and abundant mucus
Sore throat	☐0 No	☐3 Slightly sore throat	☐6 Sore dry throat with pain in swallowing	☐9 Burning pains, extremely sharp pain in swallowing
Dry throat	☐0 No	☐3 Slightly dry throat	☐6 Dry throat, sometimes with desire to drink water	☐9 Dry throat, with frequent desire to drink water
Shortness of breath	☐0 No	☐3 Mild shortness of breath	☐6 Obvious shortness of breath, which does not affect daily activity	☐9 Severe shortness of breath, with no movement ability
Wheezing	☐0 No	☐3 Occasional panting	☐6 Obvious panting, which does not affect daily activity	☐9 Severe panting, with inability to lie flat
Chest tightness	☐0 No	☐3 Slight chest tightness	☐6 Obvious chest tightness, which does not affect daily activity	☐9 Severe chest tightness, with no movement ability
Palpitation	☐0 No	☐3 Slight palpitation	☐6 Intermittent palpitation	☐9 Continuous palpitation
Dryness of the mouth	☐0 No	☐3 Mild dryness of the mouth	☐6 Dryness in the mouth, with occasional desire to drink water	☐9 Dryness in the mouth, with endless desire to drink water

Items	No	Mild	Medium	Severe
Bitter taste in mouth	☐$_0$ No	☐$_3$ Occasional bitter taste in the mouth	☐$_6$ Frequent bitter taste in the mouth	☐$_9$ Constant bitter taste in the mouth
Thirst	☐$_0$ No	☐$_3$ Dry mouth and lips	☐$_6$ Thirst	☐$_9$ Thirst with strong desire to drink water
Poor appetite	☐$_0$ No	☐$_3$ Mildly poor appetite	☐$_6$ Poor appetite	☐$_9$ No appetite
Nausea and vomiting	☐$_0$ No	☐$_3$ Nausea	☐$_6$ Vomiting	☐$_9$ Frequent vomiting; immediate vomiting of indigested food
Diarrhea	☐$_0$ No	☐$_3$ <3 times/day.	☐$_6$ 4 ~ 6 times/day.	☐$_9$ >6 times /day.
Constipation	☐$_0$ No	☐$_3$ <3 days/time.	☐$_6$ 4 ~ 6 days/time.	☐$_9$ >6 days/time.
Insomnia	☐$_0$ No	☐$_3$ Difficulty falling asleep	☐$_6$ Difficulty falling asleep, with susceptibility to be waken up	☐$_9$ Difficulty falling asleep, with susceptibility to be waken up and frequent nightmares
Tongue manifestation				

Annex 3

Picture-taking Tips for Tongue Coating

1. Natural protruding tongue. Ask the patient to stand or sit upright, with the tip of the tongue stretching downward as naturally as possible. The tongue should be kept flat, and below the level of the camera.

2. Soft and adequate lighting. The lighting should be soft and adequate. If conditions allow, make sure to take the photo with the tongue facing natural light or a fluorescent lamp.

3. Avoiding stained tongue coating. Care should be taken to avoid stained tongue coating by food or drug.

4. Covering the whole tongue. Usually, the area from below the nostril to the chin should be on the photo. The whole tongue, including the tip, the surface and the root of the tongue, should be seen.

5. The picture below for reference.

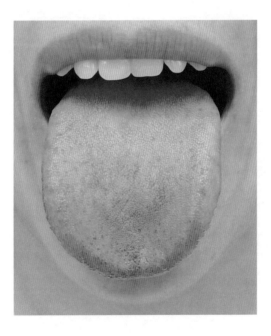

Annex 4

Acupoints Charts for Reference

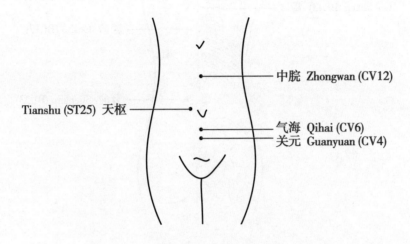

中脘 Zhongwan (CV12)

Tianshu (ST25) 天枢

气海 Qihai (CV6)
关元 Guanyuan (CV4)

Guanyuan (CV4):   on the lower abdomen, on the anterior midline, and 3 cun below the umbilicus.

Qihai (CV6):   on the lower abdomen, on the anterior midline, and 1.5 cun below the umbilicus.

Tianshu (ST25):   in the middle of the abdomen, and 2 cun lateral to the center of the umbilicus.

Zhongwan (CV12):   on the upper abdomen, on the anterior midline, and 4 cun above the umbilicus.

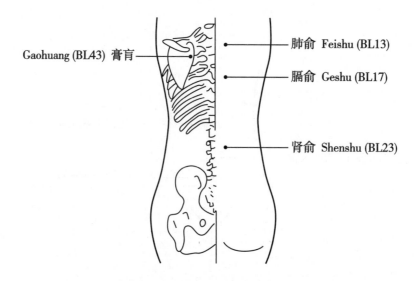

Gaohuang (BL43) 膏肓

肺俞 Feishu (BL13)

膈俞 Geshu (BL17)

肾俞 Shenshu (BL23)

Feishu (BL13):	on the back, below the 3rd thoracic spine process, and 1.5 cun lateral to the posterior midline.
Geshu (BL17):	on the back, below the 7th thoracic spine process, and 1.5 cun lateral to the posterior midline.
Shenshu (BL23):	on the waist, below the 2nd lumbar spine process, and 1.5 cun lateral to the posterior midline.
Gaohuang (BL43):	on the back, below the 4th thoracic spine process, and 3 cun lateral to the posterior midline.

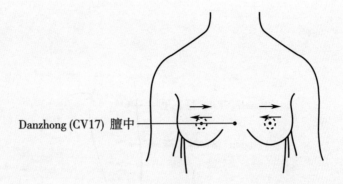

Danzhong (CV17): in the chest, on the anterior midline, at the same level as the 4th intercostal space, and on the midpoint between two nipples.

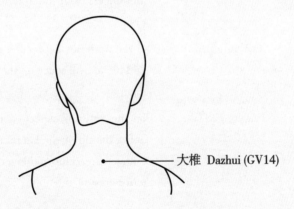

Dazhui (GV14): on the posterior midline, and in the depression below the spinous process of the 7th cervical vertebra.

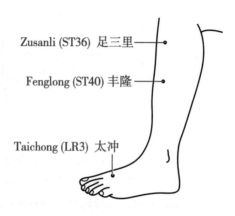

Zusanli (ST36) 足三里

Fenglong (ST40) 丰隆

Taichong (LR3) 太冲

Zusanli (ST36):	on the anterior aspect of the leg, 3 cun below Dubi (ST35), and 1 finger-breadth (midfinger) from the anterior crest of the tibia.
Taichong (LR3):	in the posterior depression of the 1st and 2nd metatarsal space on the dorsal side of the foot.
Fenglong (ST40):	on the anterior aspect of the leg, 8 cun above the tip of the lateral malleolus, and 2 finger-breadths (midfinger) from the anterior crest of the tibia.

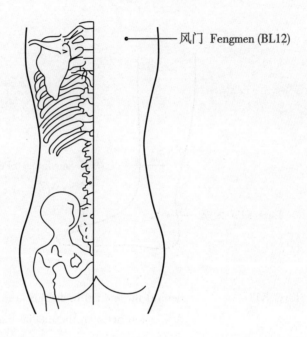

风门 Fengmen (BL12)

Fengmen (BL12):   on the back, below the 2nd thoracic spine process, and 1.5 cun lateral to the posterior midline.

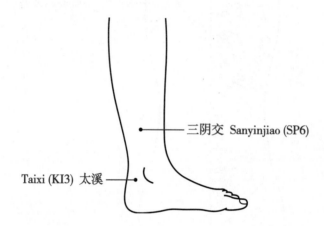

三阴交 Sanyinjiao (SP6)

Taixi (KI3) 太溪

Taixi (KI3):   behind the medial malleolus, and in the depression between the medial malleolus and tendo calcaneus.

Sanyinjiao (SP6):   on the interior aspect of the lower leg, 3 cun above the tip of the medial malleolus, and on the posterior border of the medial aspect of the tibia.

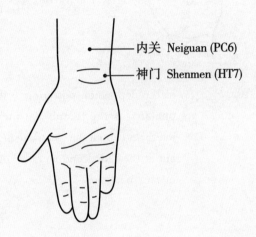

内关 Neiguan (PC6)

神门 Shenmen (HT7)

Neiguan (PC6):   on the palmar side of the forearm, 2 cun above the transverse crease of the wrist, and between the tendon palmaris longus and the tendon of flexor carpi radialis.

Shenmen (HT7):   at the wrist, at the ulnar side of the transverse crease of the wrist, and in the depression on the radial side of the tendon of flexor carpi ulnaris.

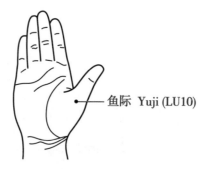

鱼际 Yuji (LU10)

Yuji (LU10):   in the depression posterior to the distal phalanx of the thumb (1st metacarpal joint), and about the red-white fleshy margin at the radial middle point of the 1st metacarpal bone.

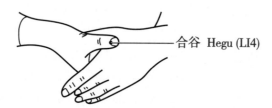

合谷 Hegu (LI4)

Hegu (LI4):   on the dorsum of the hand, between the 1st and 2nd metacarpal bones, and approximately in the middle of the 2nd metacarpal bone on the ridal side.

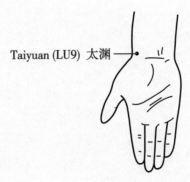

Taiyuan (LU9) 太渊

Taiyuan (LU9):   on the radial side of the palmar wrist crease, and in the depression on the radial side of radial artery.

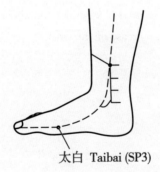

太白 Taibai (SP3)

Taibai (SP3):   on the medial aspect of the foot, in the depression poster-inferior to the 1st metatarsal bone, and at the junction of the red-white fleshy margin.

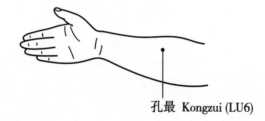

孔最 Kongzui (LU6)

Kongzui (LU6):   on the radial side of the forearm, on the line connecting Chize (LU 5) with Taiyuan (LU 9), and 7 cun above the transverse crease of the wrist.

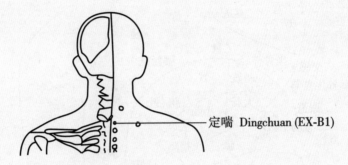

定喘 Dingchuan (EX-B1)

Dingchuan (EX-B1):   on the back, below the 7th cervical spine
process, and 0.5 cun lateral to the posteri-
or midline.

Auricular Points Diagram

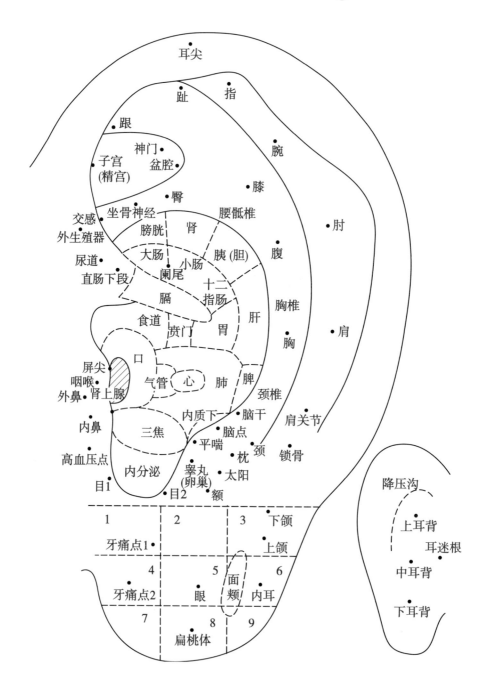

Medial surface of tragus and antitragus

耳尖：	Ear apex (HX 6, 7i)	交感：	Sympathetic (AH6a)
太阳：	Taiyang (EX-HN 5)	外生殖器：	External genitals (HX4)
枕：	Occiput (AT3)	尿道：	Urethra (HX3)
额：	Forehead (AT1)	直肠：	Rectum (HX2)
目1：	Eye 1	大肠：	Large intestine (CO7)
目2：	Eye 2	小肠：	Small intestine (CO6)
上颌：	Upper jaw	十二指肠：	Duodenum (CO5)
下颌：	Lower jaw	膀胱：	Bladder (CO9)
内耳：	Internal ear (LO6)	肾：	Kidney (CO10)
扁桃体：	Tonsil (LO7, 8, 9)	阑尾：	Appendix (CO6, 7 i)
面颊：	Cheek (LO5, 6i)	膈：	Diaphragm
眼：	Eye (LO5)	胰：	Pancreas (CO11)
牙痛点1：	Toothache Point 1	脾：	Spleen (CO13)
牙痛点2：	Toothache Point 2	肝：	Liver (CO12)
脑点：	Brain point	心：	Heart (CO15)
脑干：	Brain stem (AT3, 4i)	肺：	Lung (CO14)
颈：	Neck (AH12)	贲门：	Cardia (CO3)
颈椎：	Cervical vertebra (AH13)	胃：	Stomach (CO4)
胸：	Chest (AH10)	气管：	Trachea (CO16)
胸椎：	Thoracic vertebra (AH11)	食道：	Esophagus (CO2)
腹：	Abdomen (AH8)	皮质下：	Subcortex (AT4)
腰骶椎：	Lumbosacral vertebra (AH9)	三焦：	Triple energizer (CO17)
臀：	Gluteus (AH2)	内分泌：	Endocrine (CO18)
坐骨神经：	Sciatic nerve (AH6)	屏尖：	Tragus apex (TG1p)
膝：	Knee (AH4)	外鼻：	External nose (TG1, 2i)
趾：	Toe (AH2)	咽喉：	Pharynx larynx (TG3)
跟：	Heel (AH1)	肾上腺：	Adrenal gland (TG2p)
锁骨：	Clavicle (SF6)	内鼻：	Internal nose (TG4)
肩关节：	Shoulder joint	睾丸：	Testis (TF2)
肩：	Shoulder (SF4, 5)	卵巢：	Ovary (TF2)
肘：	Elbow (SF3)	平喘：	Antiasthma
腕：	Wrist (SF2)	降压沟：	Anti-hypertension groove
指：	Finger (SF1)	上耳背：	Upper posterior surface of ear
高血压点：	Hypertensive point	中耳背：	Middle posterior surface of ear
子宫：	Uterus (seminal vesicle)	下耳背：	Lower posterior surface of ear
神门：	Shenmen (TF4)	耳迷根：	Root of ear vagus (R2)
盆腔：	Pelvis (TF5)		

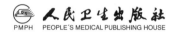

Website: http://www.pmph.com

Book Title: Diagnosis and Treatment Protocol for COVID-19: An Integrated Approach Combining Chinese and Western Medicine Recommended for International Community (Chinese-English bilingual)

面向国际的中西医结合防治新型冠状病毒肺炎诊疗建议方案（汉英对照）

Contact address: No. 19, Pan Jia Yuan Nan Li, Chaoyang District, Beijing 100021, P.R. China, phone: 8610 5978 7413, E-mail: tcy@pmph.com

First published: 2022
ISBN: 978-7-117-31517-3
Cataloguing in Publication Data:
A catalogue record for this book is available from the CIP-Database China.
Printed in The People's Republic of China

Acquisition Editor: Rao Hongmei   Li Hailing
Editor in Charge: Rao Hongmei
Book Design: Yin Yan   Ren Yi

图书在版编目（CIP）数据

面向国际的中西医结合防治新型冠状病毒肺炎诊疗建
议方案：汉英对照 / 杨明，卜海兵，朱晓新主编 . 一
北京：人民卫生出版社，2022.1
ISBN 978-7-117-31517-3

I. ①面… Ⅱ. ①杨… ②卜… ③朱… Ⅲ. ①日冕形
病毒 – 病毒病 – 肺炎 – 中西医结合疗法 – 研究 – 汉、英
Ⅳ. ①R563.105

中国版本图书馆 CIP 数据核字（2021）第 143500 号

面向国际的中西医结合防治新型冠状病毒肺炎诊疗建议方案（汉英对照）
Mianxiang Guoji de Zhong–Xi Yi Jiehe Fangzhi Xinxing Guanzhuang Bingdu
Feiyan Zhenliao Jianyi Fang'an（Han–Ying Duizhao）

主　　编	杨　明　卜海兵　朱晓新
出版发行	人民卫生出版社（中继线 010-59780011）
地　　址	北京市朝阳区潘家园南里 19 号
邮　　编	100021
印　　刷	北京顶佳世纪印刷有限公司
经　　销	新华书店
开　　本	787 × 1092　1/16　　印张：10.5　　插页：2
字　　数	150 千字
版　　次	2022 年 1 月第 1 版
印　　次	2022 年 1 月第 1 次印刷
标准书号	ISBN 978-7-117-31517-3
定　　价	88.00 元

E – mail　　pmph @ pmph.com
购书热线　　010-59787592　010-59787584　010-65264830

打击盗版举报电话：010-59787491　　E-mail：WQ @ pmph.com
质量问题联系电话：010-59787234　　E-mail：zhiliang @ pmph.com

55检